KETO RECIPES FOR WOMEN OVER 50

THE MOST DELICIOUS RECIPES TO LOSE WEIGHT AND BE MORE ENERGETIC

HANNA BLACK

Table of Contents

Introduction 8
Ketogenic Meat Recipes 12
    Cuban Beef Stew 13
    Ham Stew 15
    Delicious Veal Stew 17
    Veal And Tomatoes Dish 19
    Veal Parmesan 21
    Veal Piccata 23
    Delicious Roasted Sausage 25
    Baked Sausage And Kale 27
    Sausage With Tomatoes And Cheese 29
    Delicious Sausage Salad 31
    Delicious Sausage And Peppers Soup 33
    Italian Sausage Soup 35
Ketogenic Vegetable Recipes 37
    Amazing Broccoli And Cauliflower Cream 38
    Broccoli Stew 40
    Amazing Watercress Soup 42
    Delicious Bok Choy Soup 44
    Bok Choy Stir Fry 46
    Cream Of Celery 48
    Delightful Celery Soup 50
    Amazing Celery Stew 52
    Spinach Soup 54
    Delicious Mustard Greens Sauté 56
    Tasty Collards Greens And Ham 58
    Simple Mustard Greens Dish 62
    Collard Greens Soup 66
    Spring Green Soup 68
    Mustard Greens And Spinach Soup 70
    Roasted Asparagus 72
    Simple Asparagus Fries 74
    Amazing Asparagus And Browned Butter 76
    Asparagus Frittata 78

- Creamy Asparagus 80
- Delicious Sprouts Salad 82
- Roasted Radishes 84
- Radish Hash Browns 86
- Crispy Radishes 88
- Creamy Radishes 90
- Radish Soup 92
- Tasty Avocado Salad 94
- Avocado And Egg Salad 96
- Avocado And Cucumber Salad 98
- Delicious Avocado Soup 100
- Delicious Avocado And Bacon Soup 102
- Thai Avocado Soup 104
- Simple Arugula Salad 106
- Arugula Soup 108
- Arugula And Broccoli Soup 110

Ketogenic Meat Recipes 112
- Tasty Roasted Pork Belly 113
- Amazing Stuffed Pork 115
- Delicious Pork Chops 117
- Italian Pork Rolls 119
- Lemon And Garlic Pork 121
- Jamaican Pork 123
- Cranberry Pork Roast 124
- Juicy Pork Chops 126
- Simple And Fast Pork Chops 128
- Mediterranean Pork 130
- Simple Pork Chops Delight 132
- Spicy Pork Chops 134
- Tasty Thai Beef 136
- The Best Beef Patties 138
- Amazing Beef Roast 140
- Beef Zucchini Cups 142
- Beef And Tomato Stuffed Squash 146
- Tasty Beef Chili 148
- Glazed Beef Meatloaf 150

Delicious Beef And Tzatziki 152
Meatballs And Tasty Mushroom Sauce 154
Beef And Sauerkraut Soup 156
Ground Beef Casserole 158
Delicious Zoodles And Beef 160
Jamaican Beef Pies 162
Amazing Goulash 166
Beef And Eggplant Casserole 168
Braised Lamb Chops 170
Amazing Lamb Salad 173
Moroccan Lamb 175
Delicious Lamb And Mustard Sauce 177
Tasty Lamb Curry 179
Tasty Lamb Stew 181
Delicious Lamb Casserole 183
Amazing Lamb 185
Lavender Lamb Chops 187
Crusted Lamb Chops 189
Lamb And Orange Dressing 191
Lamb Riblets And Tasty Mint Pesto 193
Lamb With Fennel And Figs 195
Baked Veal And Cabbage 197
Delicious Beef Bourguignon 199
Roasted Beef 201
Amazing Beef Stew 203
Delicious Pork Stew 205
Delicious Sausage Stew 207
Burgundy Beef Stew 209
Duck Breast Salad 211
Turkey Pie 213
Turkey Soup 215
Baked Turkey Delight 217
Delicious Turkey Chili 219
Conclusion 221

Introduction

Do you want to make a change in your life? Do you want to become a healthier person who can enjoy a new and improved life? Then, you are definitely in the right place. You are about to discover a wonderful and very healthy diet that has changed millions of lives. We are talking about the Ketogenic diet, a lifestyle that will mesmerize you and that will make you a new person in no time.
So, let's sit back, relax and find out more about the Ketogenic diet.

A keto diet is a low carb one. This is the first and one of the most important things you should now. During such a diet, your body makes ketones in your liver and these are used as energy.
Your body will produce less insulin and glucose and a state of ketosis is induced.
Ketosis is a natural process that appears when our food intake is lower than usual. The body will soon adapt to this state and therefore you will be able to lose weight in no time but you will also become healthier and your physical and mental performances will improve.
Your blood sugar levels will improve and you won't be predisposed to diabetes.

Also, epilepsy and heart diseases can be prevented if you are on a Ketogenic diet.

Your cholesterol will improve and you will feel amazing in no time. How does that sound?

A Ketogenic diet is simple and easy to follow as long as you follow some simple rules. You don't need to make huge changes but there are some things you should know.

So, here goes!

If you are on a Ketogenic diet you can't eat:
- Grains like corn, cereals, rice, etc
- Fruits like bananas
- Sugar
- Dry beans
- Honey
- Potatoes
- Yams

If you are on a Ketogenic diet you can eat:
- Greens like spinach, green beans, kale, bok choy, etc
- Meat like poultry, fish, pork, lamb, beef, etc
- Eggs
- Above ground veggies like cauliflower or broccoli, napa cabbage or regular cabbage
- Nuts and seeds
- Cheese
- Ghee or butter
- Avocados and all kind of berries
- Sweeteners like erythritol, splenda, stevia and others that contain only a few carbs
- Coconut oil
- Avocado oil
- Olive oil

The list of foods you are allowed to eat during a keto diet is permissive and rich as you can see for yourself.
So, we think it should be pretty easy for you to start such a diet.

If you've made this choice already, then, it's time you checked our amazing keto recipe collection.

You will discover 50 of the best Ketogenic Meat and Vegetable recipes in the world and you will soon be able to make each and every one of these recipes.

Now let's start our magical culinary journey!
Ketogenic lifestyle...here we come!
Enjoy!

Ketogenic Meat Recipes

Cuban Beef Stew

A Cuban keto stew can make your day a lot better!

Preparation time: 10 minutes
Cooking time: 6 hours
Servings: 8

Ingredients:

- 2 yellow onions, chopped
- 2 tablespoons avocado oil
- 2 pounds beef roast, cubed
- 2 green bell peppers, chopped
- 1 habanero pepper, chopped
- 4 jalapenos, chopped
- 14 ounces canned tomatoes, chopped
- 2 tablespoons cilantro, chopped
- 6 garlic cloves, minced
- ½ cup water
- Salt and black pepper to the taste
- 1 and ½ teaspoons cumin, ground
- 4 teaspoons bouillon granules
- ½ cup black olives, pitted and chopped
- 1 teaspoon oregano, dried

Directions:
1. Heat up a pan with the oil over medium high heat, add beef, brown it on all sides and transfer to a slow cooker.
2. Add green bell peppers, onions, jalapenos, habanero pepper, tomatoes, garlic, water, bouillon, cilantro, oregano, cumin, salt and pepper and stir.
3. Cover slow cooker and cook on Low for 6 hours.
4. Add olives, stir, divide into bowls and serve.

Enjoy!

Nutrition: calories 305, fat 14, fiber 4, carbs 8, protein 25

Ham Stew

It's perfect for dinner tonight!

Preparation time: 10 minutes

Cooking time: 4 hours

Servings: 6

Ingredients:

- 8 ounces cheddar cheese, grated
- 14 ounces chicken stock
- ½ teaspoon garlic powder
- ½ teaspoon onion powder
- Salt and black pepper to the taste
- 4 garlic cloves, minced
- ¼ cup heavy cream
- 3 cups ham, chopped
- 16 ounces cauliflower florets

Directions:

1. In your Crockpot, mix ham with stock, cheese, cauliflower, garlic powder, onion powder, salt, pepper, garlic and heavy cream, stir, cover and cook on High for 4 hours.

2. Stir, divide into bowls and serve.

Enjoy!

Nutrition: calories 320, fat 20, fiber 3, carbs 6, protein 23

Delicious Veal Stew

No matter how busy you are, you can make the time to prepare this keto dish!

Preparation time: 10 minutes
Cooking time: 2 hours and 10 minutes
Servings: 12

Ingredients:

- 2 tablespoons avocado oil
- 3 pounds veal, cubed
- 1 yellow onion, chopped
- 1 small garlic clove, minced
- Salt and black pepper to the taste
- 1 cup water
- 1 and ½ cups marsala wine
- 10 ounces canned tomato paste
- 1 carrot, chopped
- 7 ounces mushrooms, chopped
- 3 egg yolks
- ½ cup heavy cream
- 2 teaspoons oregano, dried

Directions:

1. Heat up a pot with the oil over medium high heat, add veal, stir and brown it for a few minutes.
2. Add garlic and onion, stir and cook for 2-3 minutes more.
3. Add wine, water, oregano, tomato paste, mushrooms, carrots, salt and pepper, stir, bring to a boil, cover, reduce heat to low and cook for 1 hour and 45 minutes.
4. In a bowl, mix cream with egg yolks and whisk well.
5. Pour this into the pot, stir, cook for 15 minutes more, add more salt and pepper if needed, divide into bowls and serve.

Enjoy!

Nutrition: calories 254, fat 15, fiber 1, carbs 3, protein 23

Veal And Tomatoes Dish

Make a special dinner for your loved ones! Try this keto recipe!

Preparation time: 10 minutes

Cooking time: 40 minutes

Servings: 4

Ingredients:

- 4 medium veal leg steaks
- A drizzle of avocado oil
- 2 garlic cloves, minced
- 1 red onion, chopped
- Salt and black pepper to the taste
- 2 teaspoons sage, chopped
- 15 ounces canned tomatoes, chopped
- 2 tablespoons parsley, chopped
- 1 ounce bocconcini, sliced
- Green beans, steamed for serving

Directions:

1. Heat up a pan with the oil over medium high heat, add veal, cook for 2 minutes on each side and transfer to a baking dish.

2. Return pan to heat, add onion, stir and cook for 4 minutes.
3. Add sage and garlic, stir and cook for 1 minute.
4. Add tomatoes, stir, bring to a boil and cook for 10 minutes.
5. Pour this over veal, add bocconcini and parsley, introduce in the oven at 350 degrees G and bake for 20 minutes.
6. Divide between plates and serve with steamed green beans on the side.

Enjoy!

Nutrition: calories 276, fat 6, fiber 4, carbs 5, protein 36

Veal Parmesan

It's a very popular keto dish and you should learn how to make it!

Preparation time: 10 minutes
Cooking time: 1 hour and 10 minutes
Servings: 6

Ingredients:

- 8 veal cutlets
- 2/3 cup parmesan, grated
- 8 provolone cheese slices
- Salt and black pepper to the taste
- 5 cups tomato sauce
- A pinch of garlic salt
- Cooking spray
- 2 tablespoons ghee
- 2 tablespoons coconut oil, melted
- 1 teaspoon Italian seasoning

Directions:

1. Season veal cutlets with salt, pepper and garlic salt,

2. Heat up a pan with the ghee and the oil over medium high heat, add veal and cook until they brown on all sides.
3. Spread half of the tomato sauce on the bottom of a baking dish which you've greased with some cooking spray.
4. Add veal cutlets, then sprinkle Italian seasoning and spread the rest of the sauce.
5. Cover dish, introduce in the oven at 350 degrees F and bake for 40 minutes.
6. Uncover dish, spread provolone cheese and sprinkle parmesan, introduce in the oven again and bake for 15 minutes more.
7. Divide between plates and serve.

Enjoy!

Nutrition: calories 362, fat 21, fiber 2, carbs 6, protein 26

Veal Piccata

Make this for your loved one tonight!

Preparation time: 10 minutes
Cooking time: 15 minutes
Servings: 2

Ingredients:

- 2 tablespoons ghee
- ¼ cup white wine
- ¼ cup chicken stock
- 1 and ½ tablespoons capers
- 1 garlic clove, minced
- 8 ounces veal scallops
- Salt and black pepper to the taste

Directions:

1. Heat up a pan with half of the butter over medium high heat, add veal cutlets, season with salt and pepper, cook for 1 minute on each side and transfer to a plate.
2. Heat up the pan again over medium heat, add garlic, stir and cook for 1 minute.
3. Add wine, stir and simmer for 2 minutes.

4. Add stock, capers, salt, pepper, the rest of the ghee and return veal to pan.
5. Stir everything, cover pan and cook piccata on medium low heat until veal is tender.

Enjoy!

Nutrition: calories 204, fat 12, fiber 1, carbs 5, protein 10

Delicious Roasted Sausage

It's very easy to make at home tonight!

Preparation time: 10 minutes

Cooking time: 1 hour

Servings: 6

Ingredients:
- 3 red bell peppers, chopped
- 2 pounds Italian pork sausage, sliced
- Salt and black pepper to the taste
- 2 pounds Portobello mushrooms, sliced
- 2 sweet onions, chopped
- 1 tablespoon swerve
- A drizzle of olive oil

Directions:
1. In a baking dish, mix sausage slices with oil, salt, pepper, bell pepper, mushrooms, onion and swerve.
2. Toss to coat, introduce in the oven at 300 degrees F and bake for 1 hour.
3. Divide between plates and serve hot.

Enjoy!

Nutrition: calories 130, fat 12, fiber 1, carbs 3, protein 9

Baked Sausage And Kale

This keto dish will be ready in 20 minutes!

Preparation time: 5 minutes
Cooking time: 30 minutes
Servings: 4

Ingredients:

- 1 cup yellow onion, chopped
- 1 and ½ pound Italian pork sausage, sliced
- ½ cup red bell pepper, chopped
- Salt and black pepper to the taste
- 5 pounds kale, chopped
- 1 teaspoon garlic, minced
- ¼ cup red hot chili pepper, chopped
- 1 cup water

Directions:

1. Heat up a pan over medium high heat, add sausage, stir, reduce heat to medium and cook for 10 minutes.
2. Add onions, stir and cook for 3-4 minutes more.
3. Add bell pepper and garlic, stir and cook for 1 minute.

4. Add kale, chili pepper, salt, pepper and water, stir and cook for 10 minutes more.
5. Divide between plates and serve.

Enjoy!

Nutrition: calories 150, fat 4, fiber 1, carbs 2, protein 12

Sausage With Tomatoes And Cheese

It's a surprising and very tasty combination!

Preparation time: 10 minutes
Cooking time: 30 minutes
Servings: 4

Ingredients:

- 2 ounces coconut oil, melted
- 2 pounds Italian pork sausage, chopped
- 1 onion, sliced
- 4 sun-dried tomatoes, thinly sliced
- Salt and black pepper to the taste
- ½ pound gouda cheese, grated
- 3 yellow bell peppers, chopped
- 3 orange bell peppers, chopped
- A pinch of red pepper flakes
- A handful parsley, thinly sliced

Directions:

1. Heat up a pan with the oil over medium high heat, add sausage slices, stir, cook for 3 minutes on each side, transfer to a plate and leave aside for now.

2. Heat up the pan again over medium heat, add onion, yellow and orange bell peppers and tomatoes, stir and cook for 5 minutes.
3. Add pepper flakes, salt and pepper, stir well, cook for 1 minute and take off heat.
4. Arrange sausage slices into a baking dish, add bell peppers mix on top, add parsley and gouda as well, introduce in the oven at 350 degrees F and bake for 15 minutes.
5. Divide between plates and serve hot.

Enjoy!

Nutrition: calories 200, fat 5, fiber 3, carbs 6, protein 14

Delicious Sausage Salad

Check this out! It's very tasty!

Preparation time: 10 minutes

Cooking time: 7 minutes

Servings: 4

Ingredients:

- 8 pork sausage links, sliced
- 1 pound mixed cherry tomatoes, cut in halves
- 4 cups baby spinach
- 1 tablespoon avocado oil
- 1 pound mozzarella cheese, cubed
- 2 tablespoons lemon juice
- 2/3 cup basil pesto
- Salt and black pepper to the taste

Directions:

1. Heat up a pan with the oil over medium high heat, add sausage slices, stir and cook them for 4 minutes on each side.

2. Meanwhile, in a salad bowl, mix spinach with mozzarella, tomatoes, salt, pepper, lemon juice and pesto and toss to coat.
3. Add sausage pieces, toss again and serve.

Enjoy!

Nutrition: calories 250, fat 12, fiber 3, carbs 8, protein 18

Delicious Sausage And Peppers Soup

This keto soup will hypnotize everyone!

Preparation time: 10 minutes

Cooking time: 1 hour and 10 minutes

Servings: 6

Ingredients:

- 1 tablespoon avocado oil
- 32 ounces pork sausage meat
- 10 ounces canned tomatoes and jalapenos, chopped
- 10 ounces spinach
- 1 green bell pepper, chopped
- 4 cups beef stock
- 1 teaspoon onion powder
- Salt and black pepper to the taste
- 1 tablespoon cumin
- 1 tablespoon chili powder
- 1 teaspoon garlic powder
- 1 teaspoon Italian seasoning

Directions:

1. Heat up a pot with the oil over medium heat, add sausage, stir and brown for a couple of minutes on all sides.
2. Add green bell pepper, salt and pepper, stir and cook for 3 minutes.
3. Add tomatoes and jalapenos, stir and cook for 2 minutes more.
4. Add spinach, stir, cover and cook for 7 minutes.
5. Add stock, onion powder, garlic powder, chili powder, cumin, salt, pepper and Italian seasoning, stir everything, cover pot and cook for 30 minutes.
6. Uncover pot and cook soup for 15 minutes more.
7. Divide into bowls and serve.

Enjoy!

Nutrition: calories 524, fat 43, fiber 2, carbs 4, protein 26

Italian Sausage Soup

Everyone can make this amazing keto soup! It's so tasty and healthy!

Preparation time: 10 minutes
Cooking time: 30 minutes
Servings: 12

Ingredients:

- 64 ounces chicken stock
- A drizzle of avocado oil
- 1 cup heavy cream
- 10 ounces spinach
- 6 bacon slices, chopped
- 1 pound radishes, chopped
- 2 garlic cloves, minced
- Salt and black pepper to the taste
- A pinch of red pepper flakes, crushed
- 1 yellow onion, chopped
- 1 and ½ pounds hot pork sausage, chopped

Directions:

1. Heat up a pot with a drizzle of avocado oil over medium high heat, add sausage, onion and garlic, stir and brown for a few minutes.
2. Add stock, spinach and radishes, stir and bring to a simmer.
3. Add bacon, cream, salt, pepper and red pepper flakes, stir and cook for 20 minutes more.
4. Divide into bowls and serve.

Enjoy!

Nutrition: calories 291, fat 22, fiber 2, carbs 4, protein 17

Ketogenic Vegetable Recipes

Amazing Broccoli And Cauliflower Cream

This is so textured and delicious!

Preparation time: 10 minutes
Cooking time: 15 minutes
Servings: 5

Ingredients:

- 1 cauliflower head, florets separated
- 1 broccoli head, florets separated
- Salt and black pepper to the taste
- 2 garlic cloves, minced
- 2 bacon slices, chopped
- 2 tablespoons ghee

Directions:

1. Heat up a pot with the ghee over medium high heat, add garlic and bacon, stir and cook for 3 minutes.
2. Add cauliflower and broccoli florets, stir and cook for 2 minutes more.
3. Add water to cover them, cover pot and simmer for 10 minutes.
4. Add salt and pepper, stir again and blend soup using an immersion blender.

5. Simmer for a couple more minutes over medium heat, ladle into bowls and serve.

Enjoy!

Nutrition: calories 230, fat 3, fiber 3, carbs 6, protein 10

Broccoli Stew

This veggie stew is just delicious!

Preparation time: 10 minutes
Cooking time: 40 minutes
Servings: 4

Ingredients:

- 1 broccoli head, florets separated
- 2 teaspoons coriander seeds
- A drizzle of olive oil
- 1 yellow onion, chopped
- Salt and black pepper to the taste
- A pinch of red pepper, crushed
- 1 small ginger piece, chopped
- 1 garlic clove, minced
- 28 ounces canned tomatoes, pureed

Directions:

1. Put water in a pot, add salt, bring to a boil over medium high heat, add broccoli florets, steam them for 2 minutes, transfer them to a bowl filled with ice water, drain them and leave aside.

2. Heat up a pan over medium high heat, add coriander seeds, toast them for 4 minutes, transfer to a grinder, ground them and leave aside as well.
3. Heat up a pot with the oil over medium heat, add onions, salt, pepper and red pepper, stir and cook for 7 minutes.
4. Add ginger, garlic and coriander seeds, stir and cook for 3 minutes.
5. Add tomatoes, bring to a boil and simmer for 10 minutes.
6. Add broccoli, stir and cook your stew for 12 minutes.
7. Divide into bowls and serve.

Enjoy!

Nutrition: calories 150, fat 4, fiber 2, carbs 5, protein 12

Amazing Watercress Soup

A Chinese style keto soup sounds pretty amazing, doesn't it?

Preparation time: 10 minutes
Cooking time: 10 minutes
Servings: 4

Ingredients:

- 6 cup chicken stock
- ¼ cup sherry
- 2 teaspoons coconut aminos
- 6 and ½ cups watercress
- Salt and black pepper to the taste
- 2 teaspoons sesame seed
- 3 shallots, chopped
- 3 egg whites, whisked

Directions:

1. Put stock into a pot, mix with salt, pepper, sherry and coconut aminos, stir and bring to a boil over medium high heat.

2. Add shallots, watercress and egg whites, stir, bring to a boil, divide into bowls and serve with sesame seeds sprinkled on top.

Enjoy!

Nutrition: calories 50, fat 1, fiber 0, carbs 1, protein 5

Delicious Bok Choy Soup

You can even have this for dinner!

Preparation time: 10 minutes
Cooking time: 15 minutes
Servings: 4

Ingredients:

- 3 cups beef stock
- 1 yellow onion, chopped
- 1 bunch bok choy, chopped
- 1 and ½ cups mushrooms, chopped
- Salt and black pepper to the taste
- ½ tablespoon red pepper flakes
- 3 tablespoons coconut aminos
- 3 tablespoons parmesan, grated
- 2 tablespoons Worcestershire sauce
- 2 bacon strips, chopped

Directions:

1. Heat up a pot over medium high heat, add bacon, stir, cook until it until it's crispy, transfer to paper towels and drain grease.

2. Heat up the pot again over medium heat, add mushrooms and onions, stir and cook for 5 minutes.
3. Add stock, bok choy, coconut aminos, salt, pepper, pepper flakes and Worcestershire sauce, stir, cover and cook until bok choy is tender.
4. Ladle soup into bowls, sprinkle parmesan and bacon and serve.

Enjoy!

Nutrition: calories 100, fat 3, fiber 1, carbs 2, protein 6

Bok Choy Stir Fry

It's simple, it's easy and very delicious!

Preparation time: 10 minutes
Cooking time: 7 minutes
Servings: 2

Ingredients:

- 2 garlic cloves, minced
- 2 cup bok choy, chopped
- 2 bacon slices, chopped
- Salt and black pepper to the taste
- A drizzle of avocado oil

Directions:

1. Heat up a pan with the oil over medium heat, add bacon, stir and brown until it's crispy, transfer to paper towels and drain grease.
2. Return pan to medium heat, add garlic and bok choy, stir and cook for 4 minutes.
3. Add salt, pepper and return bacon, stir, cook for 1 minute more, divide between plates and serve.

Enjoy!

Nutrition: calories 50, fat 1, fiber 1, carbs 2, protein 2

Cream Of Celery

This will impress you!

Preparation time: 10 minutes
Cooking time: 40 minutes
Servings: 4

Ingredients:

- 1 bunch celery, chopped
- Salt and black pepper to the taste
- 3 bay leaves
- ½ garlic head, chopped
- 2 yellow onions, chopped
- 4 cups chicken stock
- ¾ cup heavy cream
- 2 tablespoons ghee

Directions:

1. Heat up a pot with the ghee over medium high heat, add onions, salt and pepper, stir and cook for 5 minutes.
2. Add bay leaves, garlic and celery, stir and cook for 15 minutes.

3. Add stock, more salt and pepper, stir, cover pot, reduce heat and simmer for 20 minutes.
4. Add cream, stir and blend everything using an immersion blender.
5. Ladle into soup bowls and serve.

Enjoy!

Nutrition: calories 150, fat 3, fiber 1, carbs 2, protein 6

Delightful Celery Soup

It's so delightful and delicious! Try it!

Preparation time: 10 minutes
Cooking time: 25 minutes
Servings: 8

Ingredients:

- 26 ounces celery leaves and stalks, chopped
- 1 tablespoon onion flakes
- Salt and black pepper to the taste
- 3 teaspoons fenugreek powder
- 3 teaspoons veggie stock powder
- 10 ounces sour cream

Directions:

1. Put celery into a pot, add water to cover, add onion flakes, salt, pepper, stock powder and fenugreek powder, stir, bring to a boil over medium heat and simmer for 20 minutes.
2. Use an immersion blender to make your cream, add sour cream, more salt and pepper and blend again.

3. Heat up soup again over medium heat, ladle into bowls and serve.

Enjoy!

Nutrition: calories 140, fat 2, fiber 1, carbs 5, protein 10

Amazing Celery Stew

This Iranian style keto stew is so tasty and easy to make!

Preparation time: 10 minutes
Cooking time: 30 minutes
Servings: 6

Ingredients:

- 1 celery bunch, roughly chopped
- 1 yellow onion, chopped
- 1 bunch green onion, chopped
- 4 garlic cloves, minced
- Salt and black pepper to the taste
- 1 parsley bunch, chopped
- 2 mint bunches, chopped
- 3 dried Persian lemons, pricked with a fork
- 2 cups water
- 2 teaspoons chicken bouillon
- 4 tablespoons olive oil

Directions:

1. Heat up a pot with the oil over medium high heat, add onion, green onions and garlic, stir and cook for 6 minutes.
2. Add celery, Persian lemons, chicken bouillon, salt, pepper and water, stir, cover pot and simmer on medium heat for 20 minutes.
3. Add parsley and mint, stir and cook for 10 minutes more.
4. Divide into bowls and serve.

Enjoy!

Nutrition: calories 170, fat 7, fiber 4, carbs 6, protein 10

Spinach Soup

It's a textured and creamy keto soup you have to try soon!

Preparation time: 10 minutes
Cooking time: 15 minutes
Servings: 8

Ingredients:

- 2 tablespoons ghee
- 20 ounces spinach, chopped
- 1 teaspoon garlic, minced
- Salt and black pepper to the taste
- 45 ounces chicken stock
- ½ teaspoon nutmeg, ground
- 2 cups heavy cream
- 1 yellow onion, chopped

Directions:

1. Heat up a pot with the ghee over medium heat, add onion, stir and cook for 4 minutes.
2. Add garlic, stir and cook for 1 minute.
3. Add spinach and stock, stir and cook for 5 minutes.

4. Blend soup with an immersion blender and heat up the soup again.
5. Add salt, pepper, nutmeg and cream, stir and cook for 5 minutes more.
6. Ladle into bowls and serve.

Enjoy!

Nutrition: calories 245, fat 24, fiber 3, carbs 4, protein 6

Delicious Mustard Greens Sauté

This is so tasty!

Preparation time: 10 minutes
Cooking time: 20 minutes
Servings: 4

Ingredients:

- 2 garlic cloves, minced
- 1 tablespoon olive oil
- 2 and ½ pounds collard greens, chopped
- 1 teaspoon lemon juice
- 1 tablespoon ghee
- Salt and black pepper to the taste

Directions:

1. Put some water in a pot, add salt and bring to a simmer over medium heat.
2. Add greens, cover and cook for 15 minutes.
3. Drain collard greens well, press out liquid and put them into a bowl.
4. Heat up a pan with the oil and the ghee over medium high heat, add collard greens, salt, pepper and garlic.

5. Stir well and cook for 5 minutes.
6. Add more salt and pepper if needed, drizzle lemon juice, stir, divide between plates and serve.

Enjoy!

Nutrition: calories 151, fat 6, fiber 3, carbs 7, protein 8

Tasty Collards Greens And Ham

This tasty dish will be ready in not time!

Preparation time: 10 minutes
Cooking time: 1 hour and 40 minutes
Servings: 4

Ingredients:

- 4 ounces ham, boneless, cooked and chopped
- 1 tablespoon olive oil
- 2 pounds collard greens, cut in medium strips
- 1 teaspoon red pepper flakes, crushed
- Salt and black pepper to the taste
- 2 cups chicken stock
- 1 yellow onion, chopped
- 4 ounces dry white wine
- 1 ounce salt pork
- ¼ cup apple cider vinegar
- ½ cup ghee, melted

Directions:

1. Heat up a pan with the oil over medium high heat, add ham and onion, stir and cook for 4 minutes.

2. Add salt pork, collard greens, stock, vinegar and wine, stir and bring to a boil.
3. Reduce heat, cover pan and cook for 1 hour and 30 minutes stirring from time to time.
4. Add ghee, discard salt pork, stir, cook everything for 10 minutes, divide between plates and serve.

Enjoy!

Nutrition: calories 150, fat 12, fiber 2, carbs 4, protein 8

Tasty Collard Greens And Tomatoes

This is just fantastic!

Preparation time: 10 minutes
Cooking time: 12 minutes
Servings: 5

Ingredients:
- 1 pound collard greens
- 3 bacon strips, chopped
- ¼ cup cherry tomatoes, halved
- 1 tablespoon apple cider vinegar
- 2 tablespoons chicken stock
- Salt and black pepper to the taste

Directions:
1. Heat up a pan over medium heat, add bacon, stir and cook until it browns.
2. Add tomatoes, collard greens, vinegar, stock, salt and pepper, stir and cook for 8 minutes.
3. Add more salt and pepper, stir again gently, divide between plates and serve.

Enjoy!

Nutrition: calories 120, fat 8, fiber 1, carbs 3, protein 7

Simple Mustard Greens Dish

Everyone can make this simple keto dish! You'll see!

Preparation time: 5 minutes
Cooking time: 15 minutes
Servings: 4

Ingredients:

- 2 garlic cloves, minced
- 1 pound mustard greens, torn
- 1 tablespoon olive oil
- ½ cup yellow onion, sliced
- Salt and black pepper to the taste
- 3 tablespoons veggie stock
- ¼ teaspoon dark sesame oil

Directions:

1. Heat up a pan with the oil over medium heat, add onions, stir and brown them for 10 minutes.
2. Add garlic, stir and cook for 1 minute.
3. Add stock, greens, salt and pepper, stir and cook for 5 minutes more.

4. Add more salt and pepper and the sesame oil, toss to coat, divide between plates and serve.

Enjoy!

Nutrition: calories 120, fat 3, fiber 1, carbs 3, protein 6

Delicious Collard Greens And Poached Eggs

This will really make everyone love your cooking!

Preparation time: 10 minutes
Cooking time: 15 minutes
Servings: 6

Ingredients:

- 1 tablespoon chipotle in adobo, mashed
- 6 eggs
- 3 tablespoons ghee
- 1 yellow onion, chopped
- 2 garlic cloves, minced
- 6 bacon slices, chopped
- 3 bunches collard greens, chopped
- ½ cup chicken stock
- Salt and black pepper to the taste
- 1 tablespoon lime juice
- Some grated cheddar cheese

Directions:

1. Heat up a pan over medium high heat, add bacon, cook until it's crispy, transfer to paper towels, drain grease and leave aside.

2. Heat up the pan again over medium heat, add garlic and onion, stir and cook for 2 minutes.
3. Return bacon to the pan, stir and cook for 3 minutes more.
4. Add chipotle in adobo paste, collard greens, salt and pepper, stir and cook for 10 minutes.
5. Add stock and lime juice and stir.
6. Make 6 holes in collard greens mix, divide ghee in them, crack an egg in each hole, cover pan and cook until eggs are done.
7. Divide this between plates and serve with cheddar cheese sprinkled on top.

Enjoy!

Nutrition: calories 245, fat 20, fiber 1, carbs 5, protein 12

Collard Greens Soup

This is a keto soup even vegetarians will love!

Preparation time: 10 minutes
Cooking time: 40 minutes
Servings: 12

Ingredients:

- 1 teaspoon chili powder
- 1 tablespoon avocado oil
- 2 teaspoons smoked paprika
- 1 teaspoon cumin
- 1 yellow onion, chopped
- A pinch of red pepper flakes
- 10 cups water
- 3 celery stalks, chopped
- 3 carrots, chopped
- 15 ounces canned tomatoes, chopped
- 2 tablespoons tamari sauce
- 6 ounces canned tomato paste
- 2 tablespoons lemon juice
- Salt and black pepper to the taste

- 6 cups collard greens, stems discarded
- 1 tablespoon swerve
- 1 teaspoon garlic granules
- 1 tablespoon herb seasoning

Directions:

1. Heat up a pot with the oil over medium high heat, add cumin, pepper flakes, paprika and chili powder and stir well.
2. Add celery, onion and carrots, stir and cook for 10 minutes.
3. Add tamari sauce, tomatoes, tomato paste, water, lemon juice, salt, pepper, herb seasoning, swerve, garlic granules and collard greens, stir, bring to a boil, cover and cook for 30 minutes.
4. Stir again, ladle into bowls and serve.

Enjoy!

Nutrition: calories 150, fat 3, fiber 2, carbs 4, protein 8

Spring Green Soup

This is a fresh spring Ketogenic soup!

Preparation time: 10 minutes
Cooking time: 30 minutes
Servings: 4

Ingredients:

- 2 cups mustard greens, chopped
- 2 cups collard greens, chopped
- 3 quarts veggie stock
- 1 yellow onion, chopped
- Salt and black pepper to the taste
- 2 tablespoons coconut aminos
- 2 teaspoons ginger, grated

Directions:

1. Put the stock into a pot and bring to a simmer over medium high heat.
2. Add mustard and collard greens, onion, salt, pepper, coconut aminos and ginger, stir, cover pot and cook for 30 minutes.

3. Blend soup using an immersion blender, add more salt and pepper, heat up over medium heat, ladle into soup bowls and serve.

Enjoy!

Nutrition: calories 140, fat 2, fiber 1, carbs 3, protein 7

Mustard Greens And Spinach Soup

This Indian style keto soup is amazing!

Preparation time: 10 minutes
Cooking time: 15 minutes
Servings: 6

Ingredients:

- ½ teaspoon fenugreek seeds
- 1 teaspoon cumin seeds
- 1 tablespoon avocado oil
- 1 teaspoon coriander seeds
- 1 cup yellow onion, chopped
- 1 tablespoon garlic, minced
- 1 tablespoon ginger, grated
- ½ teaspoon turmeric, ground
- 5 cups mustard greens, chopped
- 3 cups coconut milk
- 1 tablespoon jalapeno, chopped
- 5 cups spinach, torn
- Salt and black pepper to the taste
- 2 teaspoons ghee

- ½ teaspoon paprika

Directions:
1. Heat up a pot with the oil over medium high heat, add coriander, fenugreek and cumin seeds, stir and brown them for 2 minutes.
2. Add onions, stir and cook for 3 minutes more.
3. Add half of the garlic, jalapenos, ginger and turmeric, stir and cook for 3 minutes more.
4. Add mustard greens and spinach, stir and sauté everything for 10 minutes.
5. Add milk, salt and pepper and blend soup using an immersion blender.
6. Heat up a pan with the ghee over medium heat, add garlic and paprika, stir well and take off heat.
7. Heat up the soup over medium heat, ladle into soup bowls, drizzle ghee and paprika all over and soup.

Enjoy!

Nutrition: calories 143, fat 6, fiber 3, carbs 7, protein 7

Roasted Asparagus

It's incredibly easy and super delicious!

Preparation time: 10 minutes
Cooking time: 10 minutes
Servings: 3

Ingredients:

- 1 asparagus bunch, trimmed
- 3 teaspoons avocado oil
- A splash of lemon juice
- Salt and black pepper to the taste
- 1 tablespoon oregano, chopped

Directions:

1. Spread asparagus spears on a lined baking sheet, season with salt and pepper, drizzle oil and lemon juice, sprinkle oregano and toss to coat well.
2. Introduce in the oven at 425 degrees F and bake for 10 minutes.
   Divide between plates and serve.

Enjoy!

Nutrition: calories 130, fat 1, fiber 1, carbs 2, protein 3

Simple Asparagus Fries

These will be ready in only 10 minutes!

Preparation time: 10 minutes
Cooking time: 10 minutes
Servings: 2

Ingredients:

- ¼ cup parmesan, grated
- 16 asparagus spears, trimmed
- 1 egg, whisked
- ½ teaspoon onion powder
- 2 ounces pork rinds

Directions:

1. Crush pork rinds and put them in a bowl.
2. Add onion powder and cheese and stir everything.
3. Roll asparagus spears in egg, then dip them in pork rind mix and arrange them all on a lined baking sheet.
4. Introduce in the oven at 425 degrees F and bake for 10 minutes.
5. Divide between plates and serve them with some sour cream on the side.

Enjoy!

Nutrition: calories 120, fat 2, fiber 2, carbs 5, protein 8

Amazing Asparagus And Browned Butter

This keto dish is very delicious and it also looks wonderful!

Preparation time: 10 minutes
Cooking time: 15 minutes
Servings: 4

Ingredients:

- 5 ounces butter
- 1 tablespoon avocado oil
- 1 and ½ pounds asparagus, trimmed
- 1 and ½ tablespoons lemon juice
- A pinch of cayenne pepper
- 8 tablespoons sour cream
- Salt and black pepper to the taste
- 3 ounces parmesan, grated
- 4 eggs

Directions:

1. Heat up a pan with 2 ounces butter over medium high heat, add eggs, some salt and pepper, stir and scramble them.

2. Transfer eggs to a blender, add parmesan, sour cream, salt, pepper and cayenne pepper and blend everything well.
3. Heat up a pan with the oil over medium high heat, add asparagus, salt and pepper, roast for a few minutes, transfer to a plate and leave them aside.
4. Heat up the pan again with the rest of the butter over medium high heat, stir until it's brown, take off heat, add lemon juice and stir well.
5. Heat up the butter again, return asparagus, toss to coat, heat up well and divide between plates.
6. Add blended eggs on top and serve.

Enjoy!

Nutrition: calories 160, fat 7, fiber 2, carbs 6, protein 10

Asparagus Frittata

It's really, really tasty!

Preparation time: 10 minutes
Cooking time: 15 minutes
Servings: 4

Ingredients:

- ¼ cup yellow onion, chopped
- A drizzle of olive oil
- 1 pound asparagus spears, cut into 1 inch pieces
- Salt and black pepper to the taste
- 4 eggs, whisked
- 1 cup cheddar cheese, grated

Directions:

1. Heat up a pan with the oil over medium high heat, add onions, stir and cook for 3 minutes.
2. Add asparagus, stir and cook for 6 minutes.
3. Add eggs, stir a bit and cook for 3 minutes.
4. Add salt, pepper and sprinkle the cheese, introduce in the oven and broil for 3 minutes.
5. Divide frittata between plates and serve.

Enjoy!

Nutrition: calories 200, fat 12, fiber 2, carbs 5, protein 14

Creamy Asparagus

It's a very creamy keto dish you can try tonight!

Preparation time: 10 minutes
Cooking time: 15 minutes
Servings: 3

Ingredients:

- 10 ounces asparagus spears, cut into medium pieces and steamed
- Salt and black pepper to the taste
- 2 tablespoons parmesan, grated
- 1/3 cup Monterey jack cheese, shredded
- 2 tablespoons mustard
- 2 ounces cream cheese
- 1/3 cup heavy cream
- 3 tablespoons bacon, cooked and crumbled

Directions:

1. Heat up a pan with the mustard, heavy cream and cream cheese over medium heat and stir well.
2. Add Monterey Jack cheese and parmesan, stir and cook until it melts.

3. Add half of the bacon and the asparagus, stir and cook for 3 minutes.
4. Add the rest of the bacon, salt and pepper, stir, cook for 5 minutes, divide between plates and serve.

Enjoy!

Nutrition: calories 256, fat 23, fiber 2, carbs 5, protein 13

Delicious Sprouts Salad

This is so fresh and full of vitamins! It's wonderful!

Preparation time: 10 minutes

Cooking time: 0 minutes

Servings: 4

Ingredients:

- 1 green apple, cored and julienned
- 1 and ½ teaspoons dark sesame oil
- 4 cups alfalfa sprouts
- Salt and black pepper to the taste
- 1 and ½ teaspoons grape seed oil
- ¼ cup coconut milk yogurt
- 4 nasturtium leaves

Directions:

1. In a salad bowl mix sprouts with apple and nasturtium.
2. Add salt, pepper, sesame oil, grape seed oil and coconut yogurt, toss to coat and divide between plates.
3. Serve right away.

Enjoy!

Nutrition: calories 100, fat 3, fiber 1, carbs 2, protein 6

Roasted Radishes

If you don't have time to cook a complex dinner tonight, then try this recipe!

Preparation time: 10 minutes
Cooking time: 35 minutes
Servings: 2

Ingredients:

- 2 cups radishes, cut in quarters
- Salt and black pepper to the taste
- 2 tablespoons ghee, melted
- 1 tablespoon chives, chopped
- 1 tablespoon lemon zest

Directions:

1. Spread radishes on a lined baking sheet.
2. Add salt and pepper, chives, lemon zest and ghee, toss to coat and bake in the oven at 375 degrees F for 35 minutes.
3. Divide between plates and serve.

Enjoy!

Nutrition: calories 122, fat 12, fiber 1, carbs 3, protein 14

Radish Hash Browns

Do you want to learn how to make this tasty keto dish? Then, pay attention.

Preparation time: 10 minutes
Cooking time: 10 minutes
Servings: 4

Ingredients:

- ½ teaspoon onion powder
- 1 pound radishes, shredded
- ½ teaspoon garlic powder
- Salt and black pepper to the taste
- 4 eggs
- 1/3 cup parmesan, grated

Directions:

1. In a bowl, mix radishes with salt, pepper, onion and garlic powder, eggs and parmesan and stir well.
2. Spread this on a lined baking sheet, introduce in the oven at 375 degrees F and bake for 10 minutes.
3. Divide hash browns between plates and serve.

Enjoy!

Nutrition: calories 80, fat 5, fiber 2, carbs 5, protein 7

Crispy Radishes

It's a great keto idea!

Preparation time: 10 minutes
Cooking time: 20 minutes
Servings: 4

Ingredients:

- Cooking spray
- 15 radishes, sliced
- Salt and black pepper to the taste
- 1 tablespoon chives, chopped

Directions:

1. Arrange radish slices on a lined baking sheet and spray them with cooking oil.
2. Season with salt and pepper and sprinkle chives, introduce in the oven at 375 degrees F and bake for 10 minutes.
3. Flip them and bake for 10 minutes more.
4. Serve them cold.

Enjoy!

Nutrition: calories 30, fat 1, fiber 0.4, carbs 1, protein 0.1

Creamy Radishes

It's a creamy and tasty keto veggie dish!

Preparation time: 10 minutes
Cooking time: 25 minutes
Servings: 1

Ingredients:

- 7 ounces radishes, cut in halves
- 2 tablespoons sour cream
- 2 bacon slices
- 1 tablespoon green onion, chopped
- 1 tablespoon cheddar cheese, grated
- Hot sauce to the taste
- Salt and black pepper to the taste

Directions:

1. Put radishes into a pot, add water to cover, bring to a boil over medium heat, cook them for 10 minutes and drain.
2. Heat up a pan over medium high heat, add bacon, cook until it's crispy, transfer to paper towels, drain grease, crumble and leave aside.

3. Return pan to medium heat, add radishes, stir and sauté them for 7 minutes.
4. Add onion, salt, pepper, hot sauce and sour cream, stir and cook for 7 minutes more.
5. Transfer to a plate, top with crumbled bacon and cheddar cheese and serve.

Enjoy!

Nutrition: calories 340, fat 23, fiber 3, carbs 6, protein 15

Radish Soup

Oh my God! This tastes divine!

Preparation time: 10 minutes
Cooking time: 20 minutes
Servings: 4

Ingredients:

- 2 bunches radishes, cut in quarters
- Salt and black pepper to the taste
- 6 cups chicken stock
- 2 stalks celery, chopped
- 3 tablespoons coconut oil
- 6 garlic cloves, minced
- 1 yellow onion, chopped

Directions:

1. Heat up a pot with the oil over medium heat, add onion, celery and garlic, stir and cook for 5 minutes.
2. Add radishes, stock, salt and pepper, stir, bring to a boil, cover and simmer for 15 minutes.
3. Divide into soup bowls and serve.

Enjoy!

Nutrition: calories 120, fat 2, fiber 1, carbs 3, protein 10

Tasty Avocado Salad

This is very tasty and refreshing!

Preparation time: 10 minutes
Cooking time: 0 minutes
Servings: 4

Ingredients:

- 2 avocados, pitted and mashed
- Salt and black pepper to the taste
- ¼ teaspoon lemon stevia
- 1 tablespoon white vinegar
- 14 ounces coleslaw mix
- Juice from 2 limes
- ¼ cup red onion, chopped
- ¼ cup cilantro, chopped
- 2 tablespoons olive oil

Directions:

1. Put coleslaw mix in a salad bowl. Add avocado mash and onions and toss to coat.
2. In a bowl, mix lime juice with salt, pepper, oil, vinegar and stevia and stir well.

3. Add this to salad, toss to coat, sprinkle cilantro and serve.

Enjoy!

Nutrition: calories 100, fat 10, fiber 2, carbs 5, protein 8

Avocado And Egg Salad

You will make it again for sure!

Preparation time: 10 minutes
Cooking time: 7 minutes
Servings: 4

Ingredients:

- 4 cups mixed lettuce leaves, torn
- 4 eggs
- 1 avocado, pitted and sliced
- ¼ cup mayonnaise
- 2 teaspoons mustard
- 2 garlic cloves, minced
- 1 tablespoon chives, chopped
- Salt and black pepper to the taste

Directions:

1. Put water in a pot, add some salt, add eggs, bring to a boil over medium high heat, boil for 7 minutes, drain, cool, peel and chop them.
2. In a salad bowl, mix lettuce with eggs and avocado.

3. Add chives and garlic, some salt and pepper and toss to coat.
4. In a bowl, mix mustard with mayo, salt and pepper and stir well.
5. Add this to salad, toss well and serve right away.

Enjoy!

Nutrition: calories 234, fat 12, fiber 4, carbs 7, protein 12

Avocado And Cucumber Salad

You will ask for more! It's such a tasty summer salad!

Preparation time: 10 minutes
Cooking time: 0 minutes
Servings: 4

Ingredients:

- 1 small red onion, sliced
- 1 cucumber, sliced
- 2 avocados, pitted, peeled and chopped
- 1 pound cherry tomatoes, halved
- 2 tablespoons olive oil
- ¼ cup cilantro, chopped
- 2 tablespoons lemon juice
- Salt and black pepper to the taste

Directions:

1. In a large salad bowl, mix tomatoes with cucumber, onion and avocado and stir.
2. Add oil, salt, pepper and lemon juice and toss to coat well.
3. Serve cold with cilantro on top.

Enjoy!

Nutrition: calories 140, fat 4, fiber 2, carbs 4, protein 5

Delicious Avocado Soup

You will adore this special and delicious keto soup!

Preparation time: 10 minutes
Cooking time: 10 minutes
Servings: 4

Ingredients:

- 2 avocados, pitted, peeled and chopped
- 3 cups chicken stock
- 2 scallions, chopped
- Salt and black pepper to the taste
- 2 tablespoons ghee
- 2/3 cup heavy cream

Directions:

1. Heat up a pot with the ghee over medium heat, add scallions, stir and cook for 2 minutes.
2. Add 2 and ½ cups stock, stir and simmer for 3 minutes.
3. In your blender, mix avocados with the rest of the stock, salt, pepper and heavy cream and pulse well.
4. Add this to the pot, stir well, cook for 2 minutes and season with more salt and pepper.

5. Stir well, ladle into soup bowls and serve. Enjoy!

Nutrition: calories 332, fat 23, fiber 4, carbs 6, protein 6

Delicious Avocado And Bacon Soup

Have you ever heard about such a delicious keto soup? Then it's time you find out more about it!

Preparation time: 10 minutes
Cooking time: 10 minutes
Servings: 4

Ingredients:

- 2 avocados, pitted and cut in halves
- 4 cups chicken stock
- 1/3 cup cilantro, chopped
- Juice of ½ lime
- 1 teaspoon garlic powder
- ½ pound bacon, cooked and chopped
- Salt and black pepper to the taste

Directions:

1. Put stock in a pot and bring to a boil over medium high heat.
2. In your blender, mix avocados with garlic powder, cilantro, lime juice, salt and pepper and blend well.

3. Add this to stock and blend using an immersion blender.
4. Add bacon, more salt and pepper the taste, stir, cook for 3 minutes, ladle into soup bowls and serve.

Enjoy!

Nutrition: calories 300, fat 23, fiber 5, carbs 6, protein 17

Thai Avocado Soup

This is a great and exotic soup!

Preparation time: 10 minutes
Cooking time: 10 minutes
Servings: 4

Ingredients:

- 1 cup coconut milk
- 2 teaspoons Thai green curry paste
- 1 avocado, pitted, peeled and chopped
- 1 tablespoon cilantro, chopped
- Salt and black pepper to the taste
- 2 cups veggie stock
- Lime wedges for serving

Directions:

1. In your blender, mix avocado with salt, pepper, curry paste and coconut milk and pulse well.
2. Transfer this to a pot and heat up over medium heat.
3. Add stock, stir, bring to a simmer and cook for 5 minutes.

4. Add cilantro, more salt and pepper, stir, cook for 1 minute more, ladle into soup bowls and serve with lime wedges on the side.

Enjoy!

Nutrition: calories 240, fat 4, fiber 2, carbs 6, protein 12

Simple Arugula Salad

It's light and very tasty! Try it for dinner!

Preparation time: 10 minutes
Cooking time: 0 minutes
Servings: 4

Ingredients:

- 1 white onion, chopped
- 1 tablespoon vinegar
- 1 cup hot water
- 1 bunch baby arugula
- ¼ cup walnuts, chopped
- 2 tablespoons cilantro, chopped
- 2 garlic cloves, minced
- 2 tablespoons olive oil
- Salt and black pepper to the taste
- 1 tablespoon lemon juice

Directions:

1. In a bowl, mix water with vinegar, add onion, leave aside for 5 minutes, drain well and press.

2. In a salad bowl, mix arugula with walnuts and onion and stir.
3. Add garlic, salt, pepper, lemon juice, cilantro and oil, toss well and serve.

Enjoy!

Nutrition: calories 200, fat 2, fiber 1, carbs 5, protein 7

Arugula Soup

You have to try this great keto soup as soon as you can!

Preparation time: 10 minutes
Cooking time: 13 minutes
Servings: 6

Ingredients:

- 1 yellow onion, chopped
- 1 tablespoon olive oil
- 2 garlic cloves, minced
- ½ cup coconut milk
- 10 ounces baby arugula
- ¼ cup mixed mint, tarragon and parsley
- 2 tablespoons chives, chopped
- 4 tablespoons coconut milk yogurt
- 6 cups chicken stock
- Salt and black pepper to the taste

Directions:

1. Heat up a pot with the oil over medium high heat, add onion and garlic, stir and cook for 5 minutes.
2. Add stock and milk, stir and bring to a simmer.

3. Add arugula, tarragon, parsley and mint, stir and cook everything for 6 minutes.
4. Add coconut yogurt, salt, pepper and chives, stir, cook for 2 minutes, divide into soup bowls and serve.

Enjoy!

Nutrition: calories 200, fat 4, fiber 2, carbs 6, protein 10

Arugula And Broccoli Soup

It's one of our favorite soups!

Preparation time: 10 minutes
Cooking time: 20 minutes
Servings: 4

Ingredients:

- 1 small yellow onion, chopped
- 1 tablespoon olive oil
- 1 garlic clove, minced
- 1 broccoli head, florets separated
- Salt and black pepper to the taste
- 2 and ½ cups veggie stock
- 1 teaspoon cumin, ground
- Juice of ½ lemon
- 1 cup arugula leaves

Directions:

1. Heat up a pot with the oil over medium high heat, add onions, stir and cook for 4 minutes.
2. Add garlic, stir and cook for 1 minute.

3. Add broccoli, cumin, salt and pepper, stir and cook for 4 minutes.
4. Add stock, stir and cook for 8 minutes.
5. Blend soup using an immersion blender, add half of the arugula and blend again.
6. Add the rest of the arugula, stir and heat up the soup again.
7. Add lemon juice, stir, ladle into soup bowls and serve.

Enjoy!

Nutrition: calories 150, fat 3, fiber 1, carbs 3, protein 7

Ketogenic Meat Recipes

Tasty Roasted Pork Belly

This roasted pork belly will surprise you for sure! It's a keto recipe you must try!

Preparation time: 10 minutes
Cooking time: 1 hour and 30 minutes
Servings: 6

Ingredients:

- 2 tablespoons stevia
- 1 tablespoon lemon juice
- 1 quart water
- 17 ounces apples, cored and cut into wedges
- 2 pounds pork belly, scored
- Salt and black pepper to the taste
- A drizzle of olive oil

Directions:

1. In your blender, mix water with apples, lemon juice and stevia and pulse very well.
2. Put the pork belly in a steamer tray and steam for 1 hour.
3. Transfer pork belly to a baking sheet, rub with a drizzle of oil, season with salt and pepper and pour the apple sauce over it.

4. Introduce in the oven at 425 degrees F for 30 minutes.
5. Slice pork roast, divide between plates and serve with the applesauce on top.

Enjoy!

Nutrition: calories 456, fat 34, fiber 4, carbs 10, protein 25

Amazing Stuffed Pork

Try this keto dish really soon!

Preparation time: 10 minutes
Cooking time: 30 minutes
Servings: 4

Ingredients:

- Zest of 2 limes
- Zest from 1 orange
- Juice from 1 orange
- Juice from 2 limes
- 4 teaspoons garlic, minced
- ¾ cup olive oil
- 1 cup cilantro, chopped
- 1 cup mint, chopped
- 1 teaspoon oregano, dried
- Salt and black pepper to the taste
- 2 teaspoons cumin, ground
- 4 pork loin steaks
- 2 pickles, chopped
- 4 ham slices

- 6 Swiss cheese slices
- 2 tablespoons mustard

Directions:

1. In your food processor, mix lime zest and juice with orange zest and juice, garlic, oil, cilantro, mint, oregano, cumin, salt and pepper and blend well.
2. Season steaks with salt and pepper, place them into a bowl, add marinade you've made, toss to coat and leave aside for a couple of hours.
3. Place steaks on a working surface, divide pickles, cheese, mustard and ham on them, roll and secure with toothpicks.
4. Heat up a pan over medium high heat, add pork rolls, cook them for 2 minutes on each side and transfer them to a baking sheet.
5. Introduce in the oven at 350 degrees F and bake for 25 minutes.
6. Divide between plates and serve.

Enjoy!

Nutrition: calories 270, fat 7, fiber 2, carbs 3, protein 20

Delicious Pork Chops

These pork chops are all you need to end this day!

Preparation time: 10 minutes
Cooking time: 40 minutes
Servings: 3

Ingredients:

- 8 ounces mushrooms, sliced
- 1 teaspoon garlic powder
- 1 yellow onion, chopped
- 1 cup mayonnaise
- 3 pork chops, boneless
- 1 teaspoon nutmeg
- 1 tablespoon balsamic vinegar
- ½ cup coconut oil

Directions:

1. Heat up a pan with the oil over medium heat, add mushrooms and onions, stir and cook for 4 minutes.
2. Add pork chops, season with nutmeg and garlic powder and brown on both sides.

3. Introduce pan in the oven at 350 degrees F and bake for 30 minutes.
4. Transfer pork chops to plates and keeps warm.
5. Heat up the pan over medium heat, add vinegar and mayo over mushrooms mix, stir well and take off heat.
6. Drizzle sauce over pork chops and serve.

Enjoy!

Nutrition: calories 600, fat 10, fiber 1, carbs 8, protein 30

Italian Pork Rolls

You must pay attention and learn how to make this tasty keto dish!

Preparation time: 10 minutes
Cooking time: 20 minutes
Servings: 6

Ingredients:

- 6 prosciutto slices
- 2 tablespoons parsley, chopped
- 1 pound pork cutlets, thinly sliced
- 1/3 cup ricotta cheese
- 1 tablespoon coconut oil
- ¼ cup yellow onion, chopped
- 3 garlic cloves, minced
- 2 tablespoons parmesan, grated
- 15 ounces canned tomatoes, chopped
- 1/3 cup chicken stock
- Salt and black pepper to the taste
- ½ teaspoon Italian seasoning

Directions:

1. Use a meat pounder to flatten pork pieces.
2. Place prosciutto slices on top of each piece, then divide ricotta, parsley and parmesan.
3. Roll each pork piece and secure with a toothpick.
4. Heat up a pan with the oil over medium heat, add pork rolls, cook until they are brown on both sides and transfer to a plate.
5. Heat up the pan again over medium heat, add garlic and onion, stir and cook for 5 minutes.
6. Add stock and cook for 3 minutes more.
7. Discard toothpicks from pork rolls and return them to the pan.
8. Add tomatoes, Italian seasoning, salt and pepper, stir, bring to a boil, reduce heat to medium-low, cover pan and cook for 30 minutes.
9. Divide between plates and serve.

Enjoy!

Nutrition: calories 280, fat 17, fiber 1, carbs 2, protein 34

Lemon And Garlic Pork

You will learn how to make this tasty keto dish really soon!

Preparation time: 10 minutes
Cooking time: 30 minutes
Servings: 4

Ingredients:

- 3 tablespoons ghee
- 4 pork steaks, bone in
- 1 cup chicken stock
- Salt and black pepper to the taste
- A pinch of lemon pepper
- 3 tablespoons coconut oil
- 6 garlic cloves, minced
- 2 tablespoons parsley, chopped
- 8 ounces mushrooms, roughly chopped
- 1 lemon, sliced

Directions:

1. Heat up a pan with 2 tablespoons ghee and 2 tablespoons oil over medium high heat, add pork

steaks, season with salt and pepper, cook until they are brown on both sides and transfer to a plate.
2. Return pan to medium heat, add the rest of the ghee and oil and half of the stock.
3. Stir well and cook for 1 minute.
4. Add mushrooms and garlic, stir and cook for 4 minutes.
5. Add lemon slices, the rest of the stock, salt, pepper and lemon pepper, stir and cook everything for 5 minutes.
6. Return pork steaks to pan and cook everything for 10 minutes more.
7. Divide steaks and sauce between plates and serve.

Enjoy!

Nutrition: calories 456, fat 25, fiber 1, carbs 6, protein 40

Jamaican Pork

This simple keto dish will make you a star in the kitchen!

Preparation time: 10 minutes
Cooking time: 45 minutes
Servings: 12

Ingredients:

- 4 pounds pork shoulder
- 1 tablespoon coconut oil
- ½ cup beef stock
- ¼ cup Jamaican jerk spice mix

Directions:

1. Rub pork shoulder with Jamaican mix and place in your instant pot.
2. Add oil to the pot and set it to Sauté mode.
3. Add pork shoulder and brown it on all sides.
4. Add stock, cover pot and cook on High for 45 minutes.
5. Uncover pot, transfer pork to a platter, shred and serve. Enjoy!

Nutrition: calories 267, fat 20, fiber 0, carbs 0, protein 24

Cranberry Pork Roast

This is a keto dish that will impress you!

Preparation time: 10 minutes

Cooking time: 8 hours

Servings: 4

Ingredients:

- 1 tablespoon coconut flour
- Salt and black pepper to the taste
- 1 and ½ pounds pork loin
- A pinch of mustard, ground
- ½ teaspoon ginger
- 2 tablespoons sukrin
- 2 tablespoons sukrin gold
- ½ cup cranberries
- 2 garlic cloves, minced
- ½ lemon sliced
- ¼ cup water

Directions:

1. In a bowl, mix ginger with mustard, salt, pepper and flour and stir.

2. Add roast, toss to coat and transfer meat to a Crockpot.
3. Add sukrin and sukrin gold, cranberries, garlic, water and lemon slices.
4. Cover pot and cook on Low for 8 hours.
5. Divide on plates, drizzle pan juices on top and serve.

Enjoy!

Nutrition: calories 430, fat 23, fiber 2, carbs 3, protein 45

Juicy Pork Chops

These will be so tender and delicious!

Preparation time: 10 minutes
Cooking time: 45 minutes
Servings: 4

Ingredients:

- 2 yellow onions, chopped
- 6 bacon slices, chopped
- ½ cup chicken stock
- Salt and black pepper to the taste
- 4 pork chops

Directions:

1. Heat up a pan over medium heat, add bacon, stir, cook until it's crispy and transfer to a bowl.
2. Return pan to medium heat, add onions, some salt and pepper, stir, cover, cook for 15 minutes and transfer to the same bowl with the bacon.
3. Return pan once again to heat, increase to medium high, add pork chops, season with salt and pepper,

brown for 3 minutes on one side, flip, reduce heat to medium and cook for 7 minutes more.
4. Add stock, stir and cook for 2 minutes more.
5. Return bacon and onions to the pan, stir, cook for 1 minute more, divide between plates and serve.

Enjoy!

Nutrition: calories 325, fat 18, fiber 1, carbs 6, protein 36

Simple And Fast Pork Chops

This is going to be ready so fast!!

Preparation time: 10 minutes
Cooking time: 15 minutes
Servings: 4

Ingredients:

- 4 medium pork loin chops
- 1 teaspoon Dijon mustard
- 1 tablespoon Worcestershire sauce
- 1 teaspoon lemon juice
- 1 tablespoon water
- Salt and black pepper to the taste
- 1 teaspoon lemon pepper
- 1 tablespoon ghee
- 1 tablespoon chives, chopped

Directions:

1. In a bowl, mix water with Worcestershire sauce, mustard and lemon juice and whisk well.
2. Heat up a pan with the ghee over medium heat, add pork chops, season with salt, pepper and lemon pepper,

cook them for 6 minutes, flip and cook for 6 more minutes.
3. Transfer pork chops to a platter and keep them warm for now.
4. Heat up the pan again, pour mustard sauce you've made and bring to a gentle simmer.
5. Pour this over pork, sprinkle chives and serve.

Enjoy!

Nutrition: calories 132, fat 5, fiber 1, carbs 1, protein 18

Mediterranean Pork

This great keto dinner idea will make you feel great!

Preparation time: 10 minutes
Cooking time: 35 minutes
Servings: 4

Ingredients:

- 4 pork chops, bone-in
- Salt and black pepper to the taste
- 1 teaspoon rosemary, dried
- 3 garlic cloves, minced

Directions:

1. Season pork chops with salt and pepper and place in a roasting pan.
2. Add rosemary and garlic, introduce in the oven at 425 degrees F and bake for 10 minutes.
3. Reduce heat to 350 degrees F and roast for 25 minutes more.
4. Slice pork, divide between plates and drizzle pan juices all over.

Enjoy!

Nutrition: calories 165, fat 2, fiber 1, carbs 2, protein 26

Simple Pork Chops Delight

This is so yummy and simple to make at home!

Preparation time: 10 minutes
Cooking time: 40 minutes
Servings: 4

Ingredients:

- 4 pork chops
- 1 tablespoon oregano, chopped
- 2 garlic cloves, minced
- 1 tablespoon canola oil
- 15 ounces canned tomatoes, chopped
- 1 tablespoon tomato paste
- Salt and black pepper to the taste
- ¼ cup tomato juice

Directions:

1. Heat up a pan with the oil over medium high heat, add pork chops, season with salt and pepper, cook for 3 minutes, flip, cook for 3 minutes more and transfer to a plate.

2. Return pan to medium heat, add garlic, stir and cook for 10 seconds.
3. Add tomato juice, tomatoes and tomato paste, stir, bring to a boil and reduce heat to medium-low.
4. Add pork chops, stir, cover pan and simmer everything for 30 minutes.
5. Transfer pork chops to plates, add oregano to the pan, stir and cook for 2 minutes more.
6. Pour this over pork and serve.

Enjoy!

Nutrition: calories 210, fat 10, fiber 2, carbs 6, protein 19

Spicy Pork Chops

These spicy pork chops will impress you for sure!

Preparation time: 4 hours and 10 minutes
Cooking time: 15 minutes
Servings: 4

Ingredients:

- ¼ cup lime juice
- 4 pork rib chops
- 1 tablespoon coconut oil, melted
- 2 garlic cloves, minced
- 1 tablespoon chili powder
- 1 teaspoon cinnamon, ground
- 2 teaspoons cumin, ground
- Salt and black pepper to the taste
- ½ teaspoon hot pepper sauce
- Sliced mango for serving

Directions:

1. In a bowl, mix lime juice with oil, garlic, cumin, cinnamon, chili powder, salt, pepper and hot pepper sauce and whisk well.

2. Add pork chops, toss to coat and leave aside in the fridge for 4 hours.
3. Place pork on preheated grill over medium heat, cook for 7 minutes, flip and cook for 7 minutes more.
4. Divide between plates and serve with mango slices on the side.

Enjoy!

Nutrition: calories 200, fat 8, fiber 1, carbs 3, protein 26

Tasty Thai Beef

It will soon become your favorite keto dinner dish!

Preparation time: 10 minutes
Cooking time: 10 minutes
Servings: 6

Ingredients:

- 1 cup beef stock
- 4 tablespoons peanut butter
- ¼ teaspoon garlic powder
- ¼ teaspoon onion powder
- 1 tablespoon coconut aminos
- 1 and ½ teaspoons lemon pepper
- 1 pound beef steak, cut into strips
- Salt and black pepper to the taste
- 1 green bell pepper, chopped
- 3 green onions, chopped

Directions:

1. In a bowl, mix peanut butter with stock, aminos and lemon pepper, stir well and leave aside.

2. Heat up a pan over medium high heat, add beef, season with salt, pepper, onion and garlic powder and cook for 7 minutes.
3. Add green pepper, stir and cook for 3 minutes more.
4. Add peanut sauce you've made at the beginning and green onions, stir, cook for 1 minute more, divide between plates and serve.

Enjoy!

Nutrition: calories 224, fat 15, fiber 1, carbs 3, protein 19

The Best Beef Patties

This will be one of the best keto dishes you'll ever try!

Preparation time: 10 minutes
Cooking time: 35 minutes
Servings: 6

Ingredients:

- ½ cup bread crumbs
- 1 egg
- Salt and black pepper to the taste
- 1 and ½ pounds beef, ground
- 10 ounces canned onion soup
- 1 tablespoon coconut flour
- ¼ cup ketchup
- 3 teaspoons Worcestershire sauce
- ½ teaspoon mustard powder
- ¼ cup water

Directions:

1. In a bowl, mix 1/3 cup onion soup with beef, salt, pepper, egg and bread crumbs and stir well.

2. Heat up a pan over medium high heat, shape 6 patties from the beef mix, place them into the pan and brown on both sides.
3. Meanwhile, in a bowl, mix the rest of the soup with coconut flour, water, mustard powder, Worcestershire sauce and ketchup and stir well.
4. Pour this over beef patties, cover pan and cook for 20 minutes stirring from time to time.
5. Divide between plates and serve.

Enjoy!

Nutrition: calories 332, fat 18, fiber 1, carbs 7, protein 25

Amazing Beef Roast

It's so juicy and delicious!

Preparation time: 10 minutes
Cooking time: 1 hour and 15 minutes
Servings: 4

Ingredients:

- 3 and ½ pounds beef roast
- 4 ounces mushrooms, sliced
- 12 ounces beef stock
- 1 ounce onion soup mix
- ½ cup Italian dressing

Directions:

1. In a bowl, mix stock with onion soup mix and Italian dressing and stir.
2. Put beef roast in a pan, add mushrooms, stock mix, cover with tin foil, introduce in the oven at 300 degrees F and bake for 1 hour and 15 minutes.
3. Leave roast to cool down a bit, slice and serve with the gravy on top.

Enjoy!

Nutrition: calories 700, fat 56, fiber 2, carbs 10, protein 70

Beef Zucchini Cups

This looks so good and it tastes wonderful!

Preparation time: 10 minutes
Cooking time: 35 minutes
Servings: 4

Ingredients:

- 2 garlic cloves, minced
- 1 teaspoon cumin, ground
- 1 tablespoon coconut oil
- 1 pound beef, ground
- ½ cup red onion, chopped
- 1 teaspoon smoked paprika
- Salt and black pepper to the taste
- 3 zucchinis, sliced in halves lengthwise and insides scooped out
- ¼ cup cilantro, chopped
- ½ cup cheddar cheese, shredded
- 1 and ½ cups keto enchilada sauce
- Some chopped avocado for serving
- Some green onions, chopped for serving

- Some tomatoes, chopped for serving

Directions:
1. Heat up a pan with the oil over medium high heat, add red onions, stir and cook for 2 minutes.
2. Add beef, stir and brown for a couple of minutes.
3. Add paprika, salt, pepper, cumin and garlic, stir and cook for 2 minutes.
4. Place zucchini halves in a baking pan, stuff each with beef, pour enchilada sauce on top and sprinkle cheddar cheese.
5. Bake covered in the oven at 350 degrees F for 20 minutes.
6. Uncover the pan, sprinkle cilantro and bake for 5 minutes more.
7. Sprinkle avocado, green onions and tomatoes on top, divide between plates and serve.

Enjoy!

Nutrition: calories 222, fat 10, fiber 2, carbs 8, protein 21

Beef Meatballs Casserole

This is so special and of course, it's 100% keto!

Preparation time: 10 minutes
Cooking time: 50 minutes
Servings: 8

Ingredients:

- 1/3 cup almond flours
- 2 eggs
- 1 pound beef sausage, chopped
- 1 pound ground beef
- Salt and black pepper to taste
- 1 tablespoons parsley, dried
- ¼ teaspoon red pepper flakes
- ¼ cup parmesan, grated
- ¼ teaspoon onion powder
- ½ teaspoon garlic powder
- ¼ teaspoon oregano, dried
- 1 cup ricotta cheese
- 2 cups keto marinara sauce
- 1 and ½ cups mozzarella cheese, shredded

Directions:
1. In a bowl, mix sausage with beef, salt, pepper, almond flour, parsley, pepper flakes, onion powder, garlic powder, oregano, parmesan and eggs and stir well.
2. Shape meatballs, place them on a lined baking sheet, introduce in the oven at 375 degrees F and bake for 15 minutes.
3. Take meatballs out of the oven, transfer them to a baking dish and cover with half of the marinara sauce.
4. Add ricotta cheese all over, then pour the rest of the marinara sauce.
5. Sprinkle mozzarella all over, introduce dish in the oven at 375 degrees F and bake for 30 minutes.
6. Leave your meatballs casserole to cool down a bit before cutting and serving.

Enjoy!

Nutrition: calories 456, fat 35, fiber 3, carbs 4, protein 32

Beef And Tomato Stuffed Squash

It's always amazing to discover new and interesting dishes! This is one of them!

Preparation time: 10 minutes
Cooking time: 1 hour
Servings: 2

Ingredients:

- 2 pounds spaghetti squash, pricked with a fork
- Salt and black pepper to the taste
- 3 garlic cloves, minced
- 1 yellow onion, chopped
- 1 Portobello mushroom, sliced
- 28 ounces canned tomatoes, chopped
- 1 teaspoon oregano, dried
- ¼ teaspoon cayenne pepper
- ½ teaspoon thyme, dried
- 1 pound beef, ground
- 1 green bell pepper, chopped

Directions:

1. Place spaghetti squash on a lined baking sheet, introduce in the oven at 400 degrees F and bake for 40 minutes.
2. Cut in half, leave aside to cool down, remove seeds and leave aside.
3. Heat up a pan over medium high heat, add meat, garlic, onion and mushroom, stir and cook until meat browns.
4. Add salt, pepper, thyme, oregano, cayenne, tomatoes and green pepper, stir and cook for 10 minutes.
5. Stuff squash halves with this beef mix, introduce in the oven at 400 degrees F and bake for 10 minutes.
6. Divide between 2 plates and serve.

Enjoy!

Nutrition: calories 260, fat 7, fiber 2, carbs 4, protein 10

Tasty Beef Chili

This beef chili is so delightful! You've got to try this really soon!

Preparation time: 10 minutes
Cooking time: 8 hours
Servings: 4

Ingredients:

- 1 red onion, chopped
- 2 and ½ pounds beef, ground
- 15 ounces canned tomatoes and green chilies, chopped
- 6 ounces tomato paste
- ½ cup pickled jalapenos, chopped
- 4 tablespoons garlic, minced
- 3 celery ribs, chopped
- 2 tablespoons coconut aminos
- 4 tablespoons chili powder
- Salt and black pepper to the taste
- A pinch of cayenne pepper
- 2 tablespoons cumin, ground
- 1 teaspoon onion powder
- 1 teaspoon garlic powder

- 1 bay leaf
- 1 teaspoon oregano, dried

Directions:
1. Heat up a pan over medium high heat, add half of the onion, beef, half of the garlic, salt and pepper, stir and cook until meat browns.
2. Transfer this to your slow cooker, add the rest of the onion and garlic, but also, jalapenos, celery, tomatoes and chilies, tomato paste, canned tomatoes, coconut aminos, chili powder, salt, pepper, cumin, garlic powder, onion powder, oregano and bay leaf, stir, cover and cook on Low for 8 hours.
3. Divide into bowls and serve.

Enjoy!

Nutrition: calories 137, fat 6, fiber 2, carbs 5, protein 17

Glazed Beef Meatloaf

This will guarantee your success!

Preparation time: 10 minutes
Cooking time: 1 hour and 10 minutes
Servings: 6

Ingredients:

- 1 cup white mushrooms, chopped
- 3 pounds beef, ground
- 2 tablespoons parsley, chopped
- 2 garlic cloves, minced
- ½ cup yellow onion, chopped
- ¼ cup red bell pepper, chopped
- ½ cup almond flour
- 1/3 cup parmesan, grated
- 3 eggs
- Salt and black pepper to the taste
- 1 teaspoon balsamic vinegar
- *For the glaze:*
- 1 tablespoon swerve
- 2 tablespoons sugar-free ketchup

- 2 cups balsamic vinegar

Directions:
1. In a bowl, mix beef with salt, pepper, mushrooms, garlic, onion, bell pepper, parsley, almond flour, parmesan, 1 teaspoon vinegar, salt, pepper and eggs and stir very well.
2. Transfer this into a loaf pan and bake in the oven at 375 degrees F for 30 minutes.
3. Meanwhile, heat up a small pan over medium heat, add ketchup, swerve and 2 cups vinegar, stir well and cook for 20 minutes.
4. Take meatloaf out of the oven, spread the glaze over, introduce in the oven at the same temperature and bake for 20 minutes more.
5. Leave meatloaf to cool down, slice and serve it.

Enjoy!

Nutrition: calories 264, fat 14, fiber 3, carbs 5, protein 24

Delicious Beef And Tzatziki

You need to make sure there's enough for everyone!

Preparation time: 10 minutes

Cooking time: 15 minutes

Servings: 6

Ingredients:

- ¼ cup almond milk
- 17 ounces beef, ground
- 1 yellow onion, grated
- 5 bread slices, torn
- 1 egg, whisked
- ¼ cup parsley, chopped
- Salt and black pepper to the taste
- 2 garlic cloves, minced
- ¼ cup mint, chopped
- 2 and ½ teaspoons oregano, dried
- ¼ cup olive oil
- 7 ounces cherry tomatoes, cut in halves
- 1 cucumber, thinly sliced
- 1 cup baby spinach

- 1 and ½ tablespoons lemon juice
- 7 ounces jarred tzatziki

Directions:
1. Put torn bread in a bowl, add milk and leave aside for 3 minutes.
2. Squeeze bread, chop and put into a bowl.
3. Add beef, egg, salt, pepper, oregano, mint, parsley, garlic and onion and stir well.
4. Shape balls from this mix and place on a working surface.
5. Heat up a pan with half of the oil over medium high heat, add meatballs, cook them for 8 minutes flipping them from time to time and transfer them all to a tray.
6. In a salad bowl, mix spinach with cucumber and tomato.
7. Add meatballs, the rest of the oil, some salt, pepper and lemon juice.
8. Also add tzatziki, toss to coat and serve.

Enjoy!

Nutrition: calories 200, fat 4, fiber 1, carbs 3, protein 7

Meatballs And Tasty Mushroom Sauce

A friendly meal can turn into a feast with this keto dish!

Preparation time: 10 minutes
Cooking time: 25 minutes
Servings: 6

Ingredients:

- 2 pounds beef, ground
- Salt and black pepper to the taste
- ½ teaspoon garlic powder
- 1 tablespoon coconut aminos
- ¼ cup beef stock
- ¾ cup almond flour
- 1 tablespoon parsley, chopped
- 1 tablespoon onion flakes

For the sauce:

- 1 cup yellow onion, chopped
- 2 cups mushrooms, sliced
- 2 tablespoons bacon fat
- 2 tablespoons ghee
- ½ teaspoon coconut aminos

- ¼ cup sour cream
- ½ cup beef stock
- Salt and black pepper to the taste

Directions:

1. In a bowl, mix beef with salt, pepper, garlic powder, 1 tablespoons coconut aminos, ¼ cup beef stock, almond flour, parsley and onion flakes, stir well, shape 6 patties, place them on a baking sheet, introduce in the oven at 375 degrees F and bake for 18 minutes.
2. Meanwhile, heat up a pan with the ghee and the bacon fat over medium heat, add mushrooms, stir and cook for 4 minutes.
3. Add onions, stir and cook for 4 minutes more.
4. Add ½ teaspoon coconut aminos, sour cream and ½ cup beef stock, stir well and bring to a simmer.
5. Take off heat, add salt and pepper and stir well.
6. Divide beef patties between plates and serve with mushroom sauce on top.

Enjoy!

Nutrition: calories 435, fat 23, fiber 4, carbs 6, protein 32

Beef And Sauerkraut Soup

This beef and sauerkraut soup are so tasty!

Preparation time: 10 minutes
Cooking time: 1 hour and 20 minutes
Servings: 8

Ingredients:

- 3 teaspoons olive oil
- 1 pound beef, ground
- 14 ounces beef stock
- 2 cups chicken stock
- 14 ounces canned tomatoes and juice
- 1 tablespoon stevia
- 14 ounces sauerkraut, chopped
- 1 tablespoon gluten free Worcestershire sauce
- 4 bay leaves
- Salt and black pepper to the taste
- 3 tablespoons parsley, chopped
- 1 onion, chopped
- 1 teaspoon sage, dried
- 1 tablespoon garlic, minced

- 2 cups water

Directions:
1. Heat up a pan with 1 teaspoon oil over medium heat, add beef, stir and brown for 10 minutes.
2. Meanwhile, in a pot, mix chicken and beef stock with sauerkraut, stevia, canned tomatoes, Worcestershire sauce, parsley, sage and bay leaves, stir and bring to a simmer over medium heat.
3. Add beef to soup, stir and continue simmering.
4. Heat up the same pan with the rest of the oil over medium heat, add onions, stir and cook for 2 minutes. Add garlic, stir, cook for 1 minute more and add this to the soup.
5. Reduce heat to soup and simmer it for 1 hour.
6. Add salt, pepper and water, stir and cook for 15 minutes more.
7. Divide into bowls and serve.

Enjoy!

Nutrition: calories 250, fat 5, fiber 1, carbs 3, protein 12

Ground Beef Casserole

A friendly and casual meal requires such a keto dish!

Preparation time: 10 minutes
Cooking time: 35 minutes
Servings: 6

Ingredients:

- 2 teaspoons onion flakes
- 1 tablespoon gluten free Worcestershire sauce
- 2 pounds beef, ground
- 2 garlic cloves, minced
- Salt and black pepper to the taste
- 1 cup mozzarella cheese, shredded
- 2 cups cheddar cheese, shredded
- 1 cup Russian dressing
- 2 tablespoons sesame seeds, toasted
- 20 dill pickle slices
- 1 romaine lettuce head, torn

Directions:

1. Heat up a pan over medium heat, add beef, onion flakes, Worcestershire sauce, salt, pepper and garlic, stir and cook for 5 minutes.
2. Transfer this to a baking dish, add 1 cup cheddar cheese over it and also the mozzarella and half of the Russian dressing.
3. Stir and spread evenly.
4. Arrange pickle slices on top, sprinkle the rest of the cheddar and the sesame seeds, introduce in the oven at 350 degrees f and bake for 20 minutes.
5. Turn oven to broil and broil the casserole for 5 minutes more.
6. Divide lettuce on plates, top with a beef casserole and the rest of the Russian dressing.

Enjoy!

Nutrition: calories 554, fat 51, fiber 3, carbs 5, protein 45

Delicious Zoodles And Beef

It only takes a few minutes to make this special keto recipe!

Preparation time: 10 minutes

Cooking time: 20 minutes

Servings: 5

Ingredients:

- 1 pound beef, ground
- 1 yellow onion, chopped
- 2 garlic cloves, minced
- 14 ounces canned tomatoes, chopped
- 1 tablespoon rosemary, dried
- 1 tablespoon sage, dried
- 1 tablespoon oregano, dried
- 1 tablespoon basil, dried
- 1 tablespoon marjoram, dried
- Salt and black pepper to the taste
- 2 zucchinis, cut with a spiralizer

Directions:

1. Heat up a pan over medium heat, add garlic and onion, stir and brown for a couple of minutes.

2. Add beef, stir and cook for 6 minutes more.
3. Add tomatoes, salt, pepper, rosemary, sage, oregano, marjoram and basil, stir and simmer for 15 minutes.
4. Divide zoodles into bowls, add beef mix and serve.

Enjoy!

Nutrition: calories 320, fat 13, fiber 4, carbs 12, protein 40

Jamaican Beef Pies

This is really tasty! You must make it for your family tonight!

Preparation time: 10 minutes
Cooking time: 35 minutes
Servings: 12

Ingredients:

- 3 garlic cloves, minced
- ½ pound beef, ground
- ½ pound pork, ground
- ½ cup water
- 1 small onion, chopped
- 2 habanero peppers, chopped
- 1 teaspoon Jamaican curry powder
- 1 teaspoon thyme, dried
- 2 teaspoons coriander, ground
- ½ teaspoon allspice
- 2 teaspoons cumin, ground
- ½ teaspoon turmeric
- A pinch of cloves, ground
- Salt and black pepper to the taste

- 1 teaspoon garlic powder
- ¼ teaspoon stevia powder
- 2 tablespoons ghee

For the crust:

- 4 tablespoons ghee, melted
- 6 ounces cream cheese
- A pinch of salt
- 1 teaspoon turmeric
- ¼ teaspoon stevia
- ½ teaspoon baking powder
- 1 and ½ cups flax meal
- 2 tablespoons water
- ½ cup coconut flour

Directions:

1. In your blender, mix onion with habaneros, garlic and ½ cup water.
2. Heat up a pan over medium heat, add pork and beef meat, stir and cook for 3 minutes.
3. Add onions mix, stir and cook for 2 minutes more.
4. Add garlic, onion, curry powder, ½ teaspoon turmeric, thyme, coriander, cumin, allspice, cloves, salt, pepper, stevia powder and garlic powder, stir well and cook for 3 minutes.
5. Add 2 tablespoons ghee, stir until it melts and take this off heat.
6. Meanwhile, in a bowl, mix 1 teaspoon turmeric, with ¼ teaspoon stevia, baking powder, flax meal and coconut flour and stir.
7. In a separate bowl, mix 4 tablespoons ghee with 2 tablespoons water and cream cheese and stir.
8. Combine the 2 mixtures and mix until you obtain a dough.
9. Shape 12 balls from this mix, place them on a parchment paper and roll each into a circle.
10. Divide beef and pork mix on one half of the dough circles, cover with the other halves, seal edges and arrange them all on a lined baking sheet.

11. Bake your pies in the oven at 350 degrees F for 25 minutes.
12. Serve them warm.

Enjoy!

Nutrition: calories 267, fat 23, fiber 1, carbs 3, protein 12

Amazing Goulash

This is a keto comfort food! Try it soon!

Preparation time: 10 minutes
Cooking time: 20 minutes
Servings: 5

Ingredients:

- 2 ounces bell pepper, chopped
- 1 and ½ pounds beef, ground
- Salt and black pepper to the taste
- 2 cups cauliflower florets
- ¼ cup onion, chopped
- 14 ounces canned tomatoes and their juice
- ¼ teaspoon garlic powder
- 1 tablespoon tomato paste
- 14 ounces water

Directions:

1. Heat up a pan over medium heat, add beef, stir and brown for 5 minutes.
2. Add onion and bell pepper, stir and cook for 4 minutes more.

3. Add cauliflower, tomatoes and their juice and water, stir, bring to a simmer, cover pan and cook for 5 minutes.
4. Add tomato paste, garlic powder, salt and pepper, stir, take off heat, divide into bowls and serve.

Enjoy!

Nutrition: calories 275, fat 7, fiber 2, carbs 4, protein 10

Beef And Eggplant Casserole

These ingredients go perfectly together!

Preparation time: 30 minutes
Cooking time: 4 hours
Servings: 12

Ingredients:

- 1 tablespoon olive oil
- 2 pounds beef, ground
- 2 cups eggplant, chopped
- Salt and black pepper to the taste
- 2 teaspoons mustard
- 2 teaspoons gluten free Worcestershire sauce
- 28 ounces canned tomatoes, chopped
- 2 cups mozzarella, grated
- 16 ounces tomato sauce
- 2 tablespoons parsley, chopped
- 1 teaspoon oregano, dried

Directions:

1. Season eggplant pieces with salt and pepper, leave them aside for 30 minutes, squeeze water a bit, put

them into a bowl, add the olive oil and toss them to coat.
2. In another bowl, mix beef with salt, pepper, mustard and Worcestershire sauce and stir well.
3. Press them on the bottom of a crock pot.
4. Add eggplant and spread.
5. Also add tomatoes, tomato sauce, parsley, oregano and mozzarella.
6. Cover Crockpot and cook on Low for 4 hours.
7. Divide casserole between plates and serve hot.

Enjoy!

Nutrition: calories 200, fat 12, fiber 2, carbs 6, protein 15

Braised Lamb Chops

It's a perfect keto dish!

Preparation time: 10 minutes

Cooking time: 2 hours and 20 minutes

Servings: 4

Ingredients:

- 8 lamb chops
- 1 teaspoon garlic powder
- Salt and black pepper to the taste
- 2 teaspoons mint, crushed
- A drizzle of olive oil
- 1 shallot, chopped
- 1 cup white wine
- Juice of ½ lemon
- 1 bay leaf
- 2 cups beef stock
- Some chopped parsley for serving

For the sauce:

- 2 cups cranberries
- ½ teaspoon rosemary, chopped
- ½ cup swerve
- 1 teaspoon mint, dried

- Juice of ½ lemon
- 1 teaspoon ginger, grated
- 1 cup water
- 1 teaspoon harissa paste

Directions:
1. In a bowl, mix lamb chops with salt, pepper, 1 teaspoon garlic powder and 2 teaspoons mint and rub well.
2. Heat up a pan with a drizzle of oil over medium high heat, add lamb chops, brown them on all sides and transfer to a plate.
3. Heat up the same pan again over medium high heat, add shallots, stir and cook for 1 minute.
4. Add wine and bay leaf, stir and cook for 4 minutes.
5. Add 2 cups beef stock, parsley and juice from ½ lemon, stir and simmer for 5 minutes.
6. Return lamb, stir and cook for 10 minutes.
7. Cover pan and introduce it in the oven at 350 degrees F for 2 hours.
8. Meanwhile, heat up a pan over medium high heat, add cranberries, swerve, rosemary, 1 teaspoon mint, juice from ½ lemon, ginger, water and harissa paste, stir, bring to a simmer for 15 minutes.
9. Take lamb chops out of the oven, divide them between plates, drizzle the cranberry sauce over them and serve.

Nutrition: calories 450, fat 34, fiber 2, carbs 6, protein 26

Amazing Lamb Salad

It's a flavored salad you should try in the summer!

Preparation time: 10 minutes
Cooking time: 35 minutes
Servings: 4

Ingredients:

- 1 tablespoon olive oil
- 3 pounds leg of lamb, bone discarded and butterflied
- Salt and black pepper to the taste
- 1 teaspoon cumin, ground
- A pinch of thyme, dried
- 2 garlic cloves, minced

For the salad:

- 4 ounces feta cheese, crumbled
- ½ cup pecans
- 2 cups spinach
- 1 and ½ tablespoons lemon juice
- ¼ cup olive oil
- 1 cup mint, chopped

Directions:
1. Rub lamb with salt, pepper, 1 tablespoon oil, thyme, cumin and minced garlic, place on preheated grill over medium high heat and cook for 40 minutes, flipping once.
2. Meanwhile, spread pecans on a lined baking sheet, introduce in the oven at 350 degrees F and toast for 10 minutes.
3. Transfer grilled lamb to a cutting board, leave aside to cool down and slice.
4. In a salad bowl, mix spinach with 1 cup mint, feta cheese, ¼ cup olive oil, lemon juice, toasted pecans, salt and pepper and toss to coat.
5. Add lamb slices on top and serve.

Enjoy!

Nutrition: calories 334, fat 33, fiber 3, carbs 5, protein 7

Moroccan Lamb

Try this Moroccan keto dish as soon as you can!

Preparation time: 10 minutes
Cooking time: 15 minutes
Servings: 4

Ingredients:

- 2 teaspoons paprika
- 2 garlic cloves, minced
- 2 teaspoons oregano, dried
- 2 tablespoons sumac
- 12 lamb cutlets
- ¼ cup olive oil
- 2 tablespoons water
- 2 teaspoons cumin, ground
- 4 carrots, sliced
- ¼ cup parsley, chopped
- 2 teaspoons harissa
- 1 tablespoon red wine vinegar
- Salt and black pepper to the taste
- 2 tablespoons black olives, pitted and sliced

- 6 radishes, thinly sliced

Directions:

1. In a bowl, mix cutlets with paprika, garlic, oregano, sumac, salt, pepper, half of the oil and the water and rub well.
2. Put carrots in a pot, add water to cover, bring to a boil over medium high heat, cook for 2 minutes drain and put them in a salad bowl.
3. Add olives and radishes over carrots.
4. In another bowl, mix harissa with the rest of the oil, parsley, cumin, vinegar and a splash of water and stir well.
5. Add this to carrots mix, season with salt and pepper and toss to coat.
6. Heat up a kitchen grill over medium high heat, add lamb cutlets, grill them for 3 minutes on each side and divide them between plates.
7. Add carrots salad on the side and serve.

Enjoy!

Nutrition: calories 245, fat 32, fiber 6, carbs 4, protein 34

Delicious Lamb And Mustard Sauce

It's so rich and flavored and it's ready in only half an hour!

Preparation time: 10 minutes

Cooking time: 20 minutes

Servings: 4

Ingredients:

- 2 tablespoons olive oil
- 1 tablespoon fresh rosemary, chopped
- 2 garlic cloves, minced
- 1 and ½ pounds lamb chops
- Salt and black pepper to the taste
- 1 tablespoon shallot, chopped
- 2/3 cup heavy cream
- ½ cup beef stock
- 1 tablespoon mustard
- 2 teaspoons gluten free Worcestershire sauce
- 2 teaspoons lemon juice
- 1 teaspoon erythritol
- 2 tablespoons ghee
- A spring of rosemary

- A spring of thyme

Directions:

1. In a bowl, mix 1 tablespoon oil with garlic, salt, pepper and rosemary and whisk well.
2. Add lamb chops, toss to coat and leave aside for a few minutes.
3. Heat up a pan with the rest of the oil over medium high heat, add lamb chops, reduce heat to medium, cook them for 7 minutes, flip, cook them for 7 minutes more, transfer to a plate and keep them warm.
4. Return pan to medium heat, add shallots, stir and cook for 3 minutes.
5. Add stock, stir and cook for 1 minute.
6. Add Worcestershire sauce, mustard, erythritol, cream, rosemary and thyme spring, stir and cook for 8 minutes.
7. Add lemon juice, salt, pepper and the ghee, discard rosemary and thyme, stir well and take off heat.
8. Divide lamb chops on plates, drizzle the sauce over them and serve.

Enjoy!

Nutrition: calories 435, fat 30, fiber 4, carbs 5, protein 32

Tasty Lamb Curry

This lamb curry is going to surprise you for sure!

Preparation time: 10 minutes
Cooking time: 4 hours
Servings: 6

Ingredients:

- 2 tablespoons ginger, grated
- 2 garlic cloves, minced
- 2 teaspoons cardamom
- 1 red onion, chopped
- 6 cloves
- 1 pound lamb meat, cubed
- 2 teaspoons cumin powder
- 1 teaspoon garama masala
- ½ teaspoon chili powder
- 1 teaspoon turmeric
- 2 teaspoons coriander, ground
- 1 pound spinach
- 14 ounces canned tomatoes, chopped

Directions:

1. In your slow cooker, mix lamb with spinach, tomatoes, ginger, garlic, onion, cardamom, cloves, cumin, garam masala, chili, turmeric and coriander, stir, cover and cook on High for 4 hours.
2. Uncover slow cooker, stir your chili, divide into bowls and serve.

Enjoy!

Nutrition: calories 160, fat 6, fiber 3, carbs 7, protein 20

Tasty Lamb Stew

Don't bother looking for a Ketogenic dinner idea! This is the perfect one!

Preparation time: 10 minutes
Cooking time: 3 hours
Servings: 4

Ingredients:

- 1 yellow onion, chopped
- 3 carrots, chopped
- 2 pounds lamb, cubed
- 1 tomato, chopped
- 1 garlic clove, minced
- 2 tablespoons ghee
- 1 cup beef stock
- 1 cup white wine
- Salt and black pepper to the taste
- 2 rosemary springs
- 1 teaspoon thyme, chopped

Directions:

1. Heat up a Dutch oven over medium high heat, add oil and heat up.
2. Add lamb, salt and pepper, brown on all sides and transfer to a plate.
3. Add onion to the pot and cook for 2 minutes.
4. Add carrots, tomato, garlic, ghee, stick, wine, salt, pepper, rosemary and thyme, stir and cook for a couple of minutes.
5. Return lamb to pot, stir, reduce heat to medium low, cover and cook for 4 hours.
6. Discard rosemary springs, add more salt and pepper, stir, divide into bowls and serve.

Enjoy!

Nutrition: calories 700, fat 43, fiber 6, carbs 10, protein 67

Delicious Lamb Casserole

Serve this keto dish on a Sunday!

Preparation time: 10 minutes
Cooking time: 1 hour and 40 minutes
Servings: 2

Ingredients:

- 2 garlic cloves, minced
- 1 red onion, chopped
- 1 tablespoon olive oil
- 1 celery stick, chopped
- 10 ounces lamb fillet, cut into medium pieces
- Salt and black pepper to the taste
- 1 and ¼ cups lamb stock
- 2 carrots, chopped
- ½ tablespoon rosemary, chopped
- 1 leek, chopped
- 1 tablespoon mint sauce
- 1 teaspoon stevia
- 1 tablespoon tomato puree
- ½ cauliflower, florets separated

- ½ celeriac, chopped
- 2 tablespoons ghee

Directions:

1. Heat up a pot with the oil over medium heat, add garlic, onion and celery, stir and cook for 5 minutes.
2. Add lamb pieces, stir and cook for 3 minutes.
3. Add carrot, leek, rosemary, stock, tomato puree, mint sauce and stevia, stir, bring to a boil, cover and cook for 1 hour and 30 minutes.
4. Heat up a pot with water over medium heat, add celeriac, cover and simmer for 10 minutes.
5. Add cauliflower florets, cook for 15 minutes, drain everything and mix with salt, pepper and ghee.
6. Mash using a potato masher and divide mash between plates.
7. Add lamb and veggies mix on top and serve.

Enjoy!

Nutrition: calories 324, fat 4, fiber 5, carbs 8, protein 20

Amazing Lamb

This is a keto slow cooked lamb you will love for sure!

Preparation time: 10 minutes
Cooking time: 8 hours
Servings: 6

Ingredients:

- 2 pounds lamb leg
- Salt and black pepper to the taste
- 1 tablespoon maple extract
- 2 tablespoons mustard
- ¼ cup olive oil
- 4 thyme spring
- 6 mint leaves
- 1 teaspoon garlic, minced
- A pinch of rosemary, dried

Directions:

1. Put the oil in your slow cooker.
2. Add lamb, salt, pepper, maple extract, mustard, rosemary and garlic, rub well, cover and cook on Low for 7 hours.

3. Add mint and thyme and cook for 1 more hour.
4. Leave lamb to cool down a bit before slicing and serving with pan juices on top.

Enjoy!

Nutrition: calories 400, fat 34, fiber 1, carbs 3, protein 26

Lavender Lamb Chops

It's amazing and very flavored! Try it as soon as you can!

Preparation time: 10 minutes
Cooking time: 25 minutes
Servings: 4

Ingredients:

- 2 tablespoons rosemary, chopped
- 1 and ½ pounds lamb chops
- Salt and black pepper to the taste
- 1 tablespoon lavender, chopped
- 2 garlic cloves, minced
- 3 red oranges, cut in halves
- 2 small pieces of orange peel
- A drizzle of olive oil
- 1 teaspoon ghee

Directions:

1. In a bowl, mix lamb chops with salt, pepper, rosemary, lavender, garlic and orange peel, toss to coat and leave aside for a couple of hours.

2. Grease your kitchen grill with ghee, heat up over medium high heat, place lamb chops on it, cook for 3 minutes, flip, squeeze 1 orange half over them, cook for 3 minutes more, flip them again, cook them for 2 minutes and squeeze another orange half over them.
3. Place lamb chops on a plate and keep them warm for now..
4. Add remaining orange halves on preheated grill, cook them for 3 minutes, flip and cook them for another 3 minutes.
5. Divide lamb chops between plates, add orange halves on the side, drizzle some olive oil over them and serve.

Enjoy!

Nutrition: calories 250, fat 5, fiber 1, carbs 5, protein 8

Crusted Lamb Chops

This is easy to make and it will taste very good!

Preparation time: 10 minutes
Cooking time: 15 minutes
Servings: 4

Ingredients:

- 2 lamb racks, cut into chops
- Salt and black pepper to the taste
- 3 tablespoons paprika
- ¾ cup cumin powder
- 1 teaspoon chili powder

Directions:

1. In a bowl, mix paprika with cumin, chili, salt and pepper and stir.
2. Add lamb chops and rub them well.
3. Heat up your grill over medium temperature, add lamb chops, cook for 5 minutes, flip and cook for 5 minutes more.
4. Flip them again, cook for 2 minutes and then for 2 minutes more on the other side again.

Enjoy!

Nutrition: calories 200, fat 5, fiber 2, carbs 4, protein 8

Lamb And Orange Dressing

You will love this dish!

Preparation time: 10 minutes
Cooking time: 4 hours
Servings: 4

Ingredients:

- 2 lamb shanks
- Salt and black pepper to the taste
- 1 garlic head, peeled
- 4 tablespoons olive oil
- Juice of ½ lemon
- Zest from ½ lemon
- ½ teaspoon oregano, dried

Directions:

1. In your slow cooker, mix lamb with salt and pepper.
2. Add garlic, cover and cook on High for 4 hours.
3. Meanwhile, in a bowl, mix lemon juice with lemon zest, some salt and pepper, the olive oil and oregano and whisk very well.

4. Uncover your slow cooker, shred lamb meat and discard bone and divide between plates.
5. Drizzle the lemon dressing all over and serve.

Enjoy!

Nutrition: calories 160, fat 7, fiber 3, carbs 5, protein 12

Lamb Riblets And Tasty Mint Pesto

The pesto makes this keto dish really surprising and tasty!

Preparation time: 1 hour
Cooking time: 2 hours
Servings: 4

Ingredients:

- 1 cup parsley
- 1 cup mint
- 1 small yellow onion, roughly chopped
- 1/3 cup pistachios
- 1 teaspoon lemon zest
- 5 tablespoons avocado oil
- Salt to the taste
- 2 pounds lamb riblets
- ½ onion, chopped
- 5 garlic cloves, minced
- Juice from 1 orange

Directions:

1. In your food processor, mix parsley with mint, 1 small onion, pistachios, lemon zest, salt and avocado oil and blend very well.
2. Rub lamb with this mix, place in a bowl, cover and leave in the fridge for 1 hour.
3. Transfer lamb to a baking dish, add garlic and ½ onion to the dish as well, drizzle orange juice and bake in the oven at 250 degrees F for 2 hours.
4. Divide between plates and serve.

Enjoy!

Nutrition: calories 200, fat 4, fiber 1, carbs 5, protein 7

Lamb With Fennel And Figs

It will have a divine taste!

Preparation time: 10 minutes
Cooking time: 40 minutes
Servings: 4

Ingredients:

- 12 ounces lamb racks
- 2 fennel bulbs, sliced
- Salt and black pepper to the taste
- 2 tablespoons olive oil
- 4 figs, cut in halves
- 1/8 cup apple cider vinegar
- 1 tablespoon swerve

Directions:

1. In a bowl, mix fennel with figs, vinegar, swerve and oil, toss to coat well and transfer to a baking dish.
2. Season with salt and pepper, introduce in the oven at 400 degrees F and bake for 15 minutes.

3. Season lamb with salt and pepper, place into a heated pan over medium high heat and cook for a couple of minutes.
4. Add lamb to the baking dish with the fennel and figs, introduce in the oven and bake for 20 minutes more.
5. Divide everything between plates and serve.

Enjoy!

Nutrition: calories 230, fat 3, fiber 3, carbs 5, protein 10

Baked Veal And Cabbage

Everyone should learn how to make this wonderful dish!

Preparation time: 10 minutes
Cooking time: 40 minutes
Servings: 4

Ingredients:

- 17 ounces veal, cut into cubes
- 1 cabbage, shredded
- Salt and black pepper to the taste
- 3.4 ounces ham, roughly chopped
- 1 small yellow onion, chopped
- 2 garlic cloves, minced
- 1 tablespoon ghee
- ½ cup parmesan, grated
- ½ cup sour cream

Directions:

1. Heat up a pot with the ghee over medium high heat, add onion, stir and cook for 2 minutes.
2. Add garlic, stir and cook for 1 minute more.
3. Add ham and veal, stir and cook until they brown a bit.

4. Add cabbage, stir and cook until it softens and the meat is tender.
5. Add cream, salt, pepper and cheese, stir gently, introduce in the oven at 350 degrees F and bake for 20 minutes.
6. Divide between plates and serve.

Enjoy!

Nutrition: calories 230, fat 7, fiber 4, carbs 6, protein 29

Delicious Beef Bourguignon

It might sound a bit fancy, but it's really easy to make!

Preparation time: 3 hours and 10 minutes
Cooking time: 5 hours and 15 minutes
Servings: 8

Ingredients:

- 3 tablespoons olive oil
- 2 tablespoons onion, chopped
- 1 tablespoon parsley flakes
- 1 and ½ cups red wine
- 1 teaspoon thyme, dried
- Salt and black pepper to the taste
- 1 bay leaf
- 1/3 cup almond flour
- 4 pounds beef, cubed
- 24 small white onions
- 8 bacon slices, chopped
- 2 garlic cloves, minced
- 1 pound mushrooms, roughly chopped

Directions:

1. In a bowl, mix wine with olive oil, minced onion, thyme, parsley, salt, pepper and bay leaf and whisk well.
2. Add beef cubes, stir and leave aside for 3 hours.
3. Drain meat and reserve 1 cup of marinade.
4. Add flour over meat and toss to coat.
5. Heat up a pan over medium high heat, add bacon, stir and cook until it browns a bit.
6. Add onions, stir and cook for 3 minutes more.
7. Add garlic, stir, cook for 1 minute and transfer everything to a slow cooker.
8. Also add meat to the slow cooker and stir.
9. Heat up the pan with the bacon fat over medium high heat, add mushrooms and white onions, stir and sauté them for a couple of minutes.
10. Add these to the slow cooker as well, also add reserved marinade, some salt and pepper, cover and cook on High for 5 hours.
11. Divide between plates and serve.

Enjoy!

Nutrition: calories 435, fat 16, fiber 1, carbs 7, protein 45

Roasted Beef

It's as simple as that!

Preparation time: 10 minutes
Cooking time: 8 hours
Servings: 8

Ingredients:

- 5 pounds beef roast
- Salt and black pepper to the taste
- ½ teaspoon celery salt
- 2 teaspoons chili powder
- 1 tablespoon avocado oil
- 1 tablespoon sweet paprika
- A pinch of cayenne pepper
- ½ teaspoon garlic powder
- ½ cup beef stock
- 1 tablespoon garlic, minced
- ¼ teaspoon dry mustard

Directions:

1. Heat up a pan with the oil over medium high heat, add beef roast and brown it on all sides.

2. In a bowl, mix paprika with chili powder, celery salt, salt, pepper, cayenne, garlic powder and mustard powder and stir.
3. Add roast, rub well and transfer it to a Crockpot.
4. Add beef stock and garlic over roast and cook on Low for 8 hours.
5. Transfer beef to a cutting board, leave it to cool down a bit, slice and divide between plates.
6. Strain juices from the pot, drizzle over meat and serve.

Enjoy!

Nutrition: calories 180, fat 5, fiber 1, carbs 5, protein 25

Amazing Beef Stew

You should try this Ketogenic stew today!

Preparation time: 10 minutes
Cooking time: 4 hours and 10 minutes
Servings: 4

Ingredients:

- 8 ounces pancetta, chopped
- 4 pounds beef, cubed
- 4 garlic cloves, minced
- 2 brown onions, chopped
- 2 tablespoons olive oil
- 4 tablespoons red vinegar
- 4 cups beef stock
- 2 tablespoons tomato paste
- 2 cinnamon sticks
- 3 lemon peel strips
- A handful parsley, chopped
- 4 thyme springs
- 2 tablespoons ghee
- Salt and black pepper to the taste

Directions:

1. Heat up a pan with the oil over medium high heat, add pancetta, onion and garlic, stir and cook for 5 minutes. Add beef, stir and cook until it browns.
2. Add vinegar, salt, pepper, stock, tomato paste, cinnamon, lemon peel, thyme and ghee, stir, cook for 3 minutes and transfer everything to your slow cooker.
3. Cover and cook on High for 4 hours.
4. Discard cinnamon, lemon peel and thyme, add parsley, stir and divide into bowls.
5. Serve hot.

Enjoy!

Nutrition: calories 250, fat 6, fiber 1, carbs 7, protein 33

Delicious Pork Stew

A wonderful keto stew is all you need today!

Preparation time: 10 minutes
Cooking time: 1 hour and 20 minutes
Servings: 12

Ingredients:

- 2 tablespoons coconut oil
- 4 pounds pork, cubed
- Salt and black pepper to the taste
- 2 tablespoons ghee
- 3 garlic cloves, minced
- ¾ cup beef stock
- ¾ cup apple cider vinegar
- 3 carrots, chopped
- 1 cabbage head, shredded
- ½ cup green onion, chopped
- 1 cup whipping cream

Directions:

1. Heat up a pan with the ghee and the oil over medium high heat, add pork and brown it for a few minutes on each side.
2. Add vinegar and stock, stir well and bring to a simmer.
3. Add cabbage, garlic, salt and pepper, stir, cover and cook for 1 hour.
4. Add carrots and green onions, stir and cook for 15 minutes more.
5. Add whipping cream, stir for 1 minute, divide between plates and serve.

Enjoy!

Nutrition: calories 400, fat 25, fiber 3, carbs 6, protein 43

Delicious Sausage Stew

We recommend you to try this stew if you are on a keto diet!

Preparation time: 10 minutes
Cooking time: 20 minutes
Servings: 9

Ingredients:

- 1 pound smoked sausage, sliced
- 1 green bell pepper, chopped
- 2 yellow onions, chopped
- Salt and black pepper to the taste
- 1 cup parsley, chopped
- 8 green onions, chopped
- ¼ cup avocado oil
- 1 cup beef stock
- 6 garlic cloves
- 28 ounces canned tomatoes, chopped
- 16 ounces okra, chopped
- 8 ounces tomato sauce
- 2 tablespoons coconut aminos
- 1 tablespoon gluten free hot sauce

Directions:
1. Heat up a pot with the oil over medium high heat, add sausages, stir and cook for 2 minutes.
2. Add onion, bell pepper, green onions, parsley, salt and pepper, stir and cook for 2 minutes more.
3. Add stock, garlic, tomatoes, okra, tomato sauce, coconut aminos and hot sauce, stir, bring to a simmer and cook for 15 minutes.
4. Add more salt and pepper, stir, divide into bowls and serve.

Enjoy!

Nutrition: calories 274, fat 20, fiber 4, carbs 7, protein 10

Burgundy Beef Stew

It's time to learn how to make a special keto stew for your loved ones!

Preparation time: 10 minutes
Cooking time: 3 hours
Servings: 7

Ingredients:

- 2 pounds beef chuck roast, cubed
- 15 ounces canned tomatoes, chopped
- 4 carrots, chopped
- Salt and black pepper to the taste
- ½ pounds mushrooms, sliced
- 2 celery ribs, chopped
- 2 yellow onions, chopped
- 1 cup beef stock
- 1 tablespoon thyme, chopped
- ½ teaspoon mustard powder
- 3 tablespoons almond flour
- 1 cup water

Directions:

1. Heat up an oven proof pot over medium high heat, add beef cubes, stir and brown them for a couple of minutes on each side.
2. Add tomatoes, mushrooms, onions, carrots, celery, salt, pepper mustard, stock and thyme and stir.
3. In a bowl mix water with flour and stir well. Add this to the pot, stir well, introduce in the oven and bake at 325 degrees F for 3 hours.
4. Stir every half an hour.
5. Divide into bowls and serve.

Enjoy!

Nutrition: calories 275, fat 13, fiber 4, carbs 7, protein 28

Duck Breast Salad

It's a tasty salad with a delicious vinaigrette!

Preparation time: 10 minutes
Cooking time: 15 minutes
Servings: 4

Ingredients:

- 1 tablespoon swerve
- 1 shallot, chopped
- ¼ cup red vinegar
- ¼ cup olive oil
- ¼ cup water
- ¾ cup raspberries
- 1 tablespoon Dijon mustard
- Salt and black pepper to the taste

For the salad:

- 10 ounces baby spinach
- 2 medium duck breasts, boneless
- 4 ounces goat cheese, crumbled
- Salt and black pepper to the taste
- ½ pint raspberries
- ½ cup pecans halves

Directions:

1. In your blender, mix swerve with shallot, vinegar, water, oil, ¾ cup raspberries, mustard, salt and pepper and blend very well.
2. Strain this, put into a bowl and leave aside.
3. Score duck breast, season with salt and pepper and place skin side down into a pan heated up over medium high heat.
4. Cook for 8 minutes, flip and cook for 5 minutes more.
5. Divide spinach on plates, sprinkle goat cheese, pecan halves and ½ pint raspberries.
6. Slice duck breasts and add on top of raspberries.
7. Drizzle the raspberries vinaigrette on top and serve.

Enjoy!

Nutrition: calories 455, fat 40, fiber 4, carbs 6, protein 18

Turkey Pie

It's a great way to end your day!

Preparation time: 10 minutes
Cooking time: 40 minutes
Servings: 6
Ingredients:

- 2 cups turkey stock
- 1 cup turkey meat, cooked and shredded
- Salt and black pepper to the taste
- 1 teaspoon thyme, chopped
- ½ cup kale, chopped
- ½ cup butternut squash, peeled and chopped
- ½ cup cheddar cheese, shredded
- ¼ teaspoon paprika
- ¼ teaspoon garlic powder
- ¼ teaspoon xanthan gum
- Cooking spray

For the crust:

- ¼ cup ghee
- ¼ teaspoon xanthan gum
- 2 cups almond flour
- A pinch of salt

- 1 egg
- ¼ cup cheddar cheese

Directions:
1. Heat up a pot with the stock over medium heat.
2. Add squash and turkey meat, stir and cook for 10 minutes.
3. Add garlic powder, kale, thyme, paprika, salt, pepper and ½ cup cheddar cheese and stir well.
4. In a bowl, mix ¼ teaspoon xanthan gum with ½ cup stock from the pot, stir well and add everything to the pot.
5. Take off heat and leave aside for now.
6. In a bowl, mix flour with ¼ teaspoon xanthan gum and a pinch of salt and stir.
7. Add ghee, egg and ¼ cup cheddar cheese and stir everything until you obtain your pie crust dough.
8. Shape a ball and keep in the fridge for now.
9. Spray a baking dish with cooking spray and spread pie filling on the bottom.
10. Transfer dough to a working surface, roll into a circle and top filling with this.
11. Press well and seal edges, introduce in the oven at 350 degrees F and bake for 35 minutes.
12. Leave the pie to cool down a bit and serve.

Nutrition: calories 320, fat 23, fiber 8, carbs 6, protein 16

Turkey Soup

It's a very comforting and rich soup!

Preparation time: 10 minutes
Cooking time: 30 minutes
Servings: 4

Ingredients:

- 3 celery stalks, chopped
- 1 yellow onion, chopped
- 1 tablespoon ghee
- 6 cups turkey stock
- Salt and black pepper to the taste
- ¼ cup parsley, chopped
- 3 cups baked spaghetti squash, chopped
- 3 cups turkey, cooked and shredded

Directions:

1. Heat up a pot with the ghee over medium high heat, add celery and onion, stir and cook for 5 minutes.
2. Add parsley, stock, turkey meat, salt and pepper, stir and cook for 20 minutes.

3. Add spaghetti squash, stir and cook turkey soup for 10 minutes more.
4. Divide into bowls and serve.

Enjoy!

Nutrition: calories 150, fat 4, fiber 1, carbs 3, protein 10

Baked Turkey Delight

Try it soon! You will make it a second time as well!

Preparation time: 10 minutes
Cooking time: 45 minutes
Servings: 8

Ingredients:

- 4 cups zucchinis, cut with a spiralizer
- 1 egg, whisked
- 3 cups cabbage, shredded
- 3 cups turkey meat, cooked and shredded
- ½ cup turkey stock
- ½ cup cream cheese
- 1 teaspoon poultry seasoning
- 2 cup cheddar cheese, grated
- ½ cup parmesan cheese, grated
- Salt and black pepper to the taste
- ¼ teaspoon garlic powder

Directions:

1. Heat up a pan with the stock over medium-low heat.

2. Add egg, cream, parmesan, cheddar cheese, salt, pepper, poultry seasoning and garlic powder, stir and bring to a gentle simmer.
3. Add turkey meat and cabbage, stir and take off heat.
4. Place zucchini noodles in a baking dish, add some salt and pepper, pour turkey mix and spread.
5. Cover with tin foil, introduce in the oven at 400 degrees F and bake for 35 minutes.
6. Leave aside to cool down a bit before serving.

Enjoy!

Nutrition: calories 240, fat 15, fiber 1, carbs 3, protein 25

Delicious Turkey Chili

This great keto dish is perfect for a cold and rainy day!

Preparation time: 10 minutes
Cooking time: 20 minutes
Servings: 8

Ingredients:

- 4 cups turkey meat, cooked and shredded
- 2 cups squash, chopped
- 6 cups chicken stock
- Salt and black pepper to the taste
- 1 tablespoon canned chipotle peppers, chopped
- ½ teaspoon garlic powder
- ½ cup salsa verde
- 1 teaspoon coriander, ground
- 2 teaspoons cumin, ground
- ¼ cup sour cream
- 1 tablespoon cilantro, chopped

Directions:

1. Heat up a pan with the stock over medium heat.
2. Add squash, stir and cook for 10 minutes.

3. Add turkey, chipotles, garlic powder, salsa verde, cumin, coriander, salt and pepper, stir and cook for 10 minutes.
4. Add sour cream, stir, take off heat and divide into bowls.
5. Top with some chopped cilantro and serve.

Enjoy!

Nutrition: calories 154, fat 5, fiber 3, carbs 2, protein 27

Conclusion

This is really a life changing cookbook. It shows you everything you need to know about the Ketogenic diet and it helps you get started. You now know some of the best and most popular Ketogenic recipes in the world.

We have something for everyone's taste!

So, don't hesitate too much and start your new life as a follower of the Ketogenic diet!

Get your hands on this special recipes collection and start cooking in this new, exciting and healthy way!

Have a lot of fun and enjoy your Ketogenic diet!

www.ingramcontent.com/pod-product-compliance
Lightning Source LLC
Chambersburg PA
CBHW071816080526
44589CB00012B/809